LOSING MY SISTER

Also by Judy Goldman

FICTION

Early Leaving
The Slow Way Back

POETRY

Wanting to Know the End
Holding Back Winter

LOSING MY SISTER

a memoir by *Judy Goldman*

JOHN F. BLAIR, PUBLISHER
Winston-Salem, North Carolina

Published by
JOHN F. BLAIR,
P U B L I S H E R
1406 Plaza Drive
Winston-Salem, North Carolina 27103
www.blairpub.com

COVER PHOTOGRAPH
Judy and Brenda, 1944

Jacket design by Laurie Goldman Smithwick
Book design by Debra Long Hampton

Library of Congress Cataloging-in-Publication Data

Goldman, Judy.
  Losing my sister : a memoir / by Judy Goldman.
      p.   cm.
  ISBN 978-0-89587-583-9 (alk. paper) — ISBN 978-0-89587-584-6 (ebook)
1. Goldman, Judy—Family relationships. 2. Women novelists, American—Biog-
raphy. 3. Breast—Cancer—Patients—Biography. I. Title.
  PS3557.O3688Z46 2012
  813'.54—dc23
  [B]
                          2012021309

10 9 8 7 6 5 4 3 2 1

For Henry

For Laurie and Bob,
Lucy and Zoe

For Mike and Brooke,
Tess and Benjamin

For Donald

In loving memory of Brenda, my parents, and Mattie

Acknowledgments

I gratefully acknowledge the editors of the following publications, in which portions of this book originally appeared, sometimes in different form:

Real Simple magazine
The Southern Review
Shenandoah
Black Warrior Review
The Charlotte Observer
Wanting to Know the End

Portions also appeared in the following anthologies:

Claiming the Spirit Within: A Sourcebook of Women's Poetry (Beacon Press)
Ladies, Start Your Engines: Women Writers on Cars and the Road (Faber and Faber)
Here's to the Land: 60th Anniversary Anthology of the North Carolina Poetry Society
Luck: A Collection of Facts, Fiction, Incantations & Verse (Lorimer Press)

A portion also appeared in the following online journal:

Drafthorse: A Lit Journal of Work and No Work

I read portions of this book as personal commentaries on WFAE-FM, the NPR affiliate in Charlotte, North Carolina, and on WUNC-FM, the NPR affiliate in Chapel Hill, North Carolina.

Huge gratitude for many different things: Abigail DeWitt, my breakfast group (Bobbie Campbell, Mary Hunter Daly, Ann Haskell, Laurie Johnston, Clarissa Porter, Dannye Powell), Judy Pera, Marilyn Perlman, Ruth Cohen, Debbie Rubin, Mary Fenster, Paula Reckson, Darnell Arnoult, Georgann Eubanks, Dwight Allen, Dana Sachs, Peggy Payne, Christina Baker Kline, Mike Chitwood, Paul Austin, Betsy Thorpe, Charla Muller, Claire Bateman, Lindsay Reckson, and Stephanie Whetstone.

Equally huge gratitude: my magnificent, enthusiastic, and very smart agent, Amy Rennert, and the exceptionally talented, hardworking, and lovely folks at John F. Blair, Publisher: Carolyn Sakowski, Steve Kirk, Angela Harwood, Debra Long Hampton, and Brooke Csuka.

Also, gratitude to my daughter, Laurie Goldman Smithwick, for a cover design that brings tears to my eyes.

❧

The names of some people in this book have been changed. Details have been re-created from journal notes, recent interviews, and memory. Throughout the six years I was working on this memoir, I struggled with the question: *Am I taking liberties? Embellishing?* And, of course, the big question: do I even have the right to tell this story? In fact, the act of remembering is inevitably an act of revision. All I could do was keep my eye on one goal: try to tell the truth, as I know it.

LOSING MY SISTER

Opening Words

It's 1992 and I'm soaping my breasts in the shower so I can check for lumps. The first time a doctor told me I should do periodic breast exams, I laughed and said, "That'll be easy. It should take about a minute!"

But I'm feeling something in my left breast. More soap. Lather. Stand up straighter. This thing is not just a lump. It's what you'd call a mass.

In bed, before sleep, I guide my husband's sweet and careful hand to the spot.

"Right here," I say. "Feel it?"

"I do," Henry says.

I can't help noticing the way his dark, heavy eyebrows squeeze together in the middle of his forehead, the funny way his mouth is twisting to the side. I hate telling him. Not just because he's going to be worried, but because saying the words out loud makes them real.

Next morning, I call two people: My doctor. And my sister. Brenda, three years older, is the person I want to tell if something is wrong. She's practical, clearheaded. She knows what to do. What to think. Well, the real story is, she knows what *I* should do, what *I* should think. When Brenda says it, I believe it.

But she has her own news.

She's just had a routine mammogram—*she* was getting ready to call me!—and they discovered calcifications in her breast.

"Not exactly a tumor. More like sprinkles," she explains. "But it could be breast cancer."

Our doctors refer each of us to a surgeon. The same surgeon. My appointment is the day after hers.

I'll soon begin writing a novel in which the two main characters, Mickey and Thea, are based loosely on Brenda and me. In the book, each sister discovers a lump in her breast.

After the book is published, I'll give a reading in one of those bookstores with hardwood floors and deep, upholstered wing chairs. A woman in the audience will say that she finds the situation with the two sisters and their biopsies hard to believe.

"What are the chances of two sisters having tumors in their breasts at the same time?" she'll ask, leaning forward in the chair, wrapping her arms around herself, satisfied to be *on* to me, to expose my insubstantial grasp of reality.

Students in fiction workshops are always defending their far-fetched plot twists by insisting, *But it really happened that way.*

My job as teacher is to say, *It doesn't matter. What you write has to seem believable to the reader.*

"But it really happened that way," I'll hear myself telling the woman.

Brenda sees the surgeon, doesn't like his abrupt manner. "I know he's used to dealing with patients who are asleep," she tells me, that closed tone of voice, "but I'm not going to put up with his rudeness."

The next day, I see him. I mention that he saw my sister. He immediately lets me know that *he* knows she was not exactly thrilled with him. He says to me, "You make sure your sister has those calcifications biopsied. It doesn't matter whether I'm the surgeon or not. She needs a needle biopsy. As quickly as possible."

Then he examines my breasts, his eyes gliding across my face until he finally focuses on the wall behind me. All the while, he's kneading.

But then he spends more time talking about Brenda's situation than mine. I think he knows something. Which makes my mouth go dry. I'm suddenly more worried about her than me. Being the younger sister, I've always thought of her as more important. It's not a problem. Just the way it is. In my mind, she's Technicolor and I'm black-and-white. She's an entrée. I'm a side dish.

Brenda finds a different surgeon. In an uncharacteristically independent move, I stay with Dr. Abrupt.

Our biopsies take place one day apart.

We both wait for the pathology reports.

Mine is benign.

Hers, malignant.

Which is a capsule image of the two of us. I'm that prim type of person you could call benign. And Brenda—she is certainly not malignant, but she is *tough*.

Our pathology reports are symbolic in another way: they're indelible examples of my perennial good luck and her bad.

In small and large ways, Brenda's life has not been easy. She started wearing glasses in the fifth grade, had to wear braces for years. She matured late; her friends matured early; they dropped her in the eighth grade, did not take her back until the tenth. She didn't have a boyfriend till freshman year in college. My life has been different. My eyes were fine, teeth straight. I started dating in the sixth grade and remained close with my girlfriends throughout. She gave birth to four boys in six years, had three in diapers at the same time. I had a girl and a boy, spaced three easy years apart. Barely three months after her first baby was born, she suffered terrible injuries in a car accident.

And all this pales in comparison to what she'll go through later.

For now, though, this feels like an extreme situation, an intense danger, a watershed. She and I react the only ways we know. She stays strong. I worry. I'm with her for the duration—the mastectomy, her recuperation in the hospital, recuperation at home.

Months later, I go with her to the plastic surgeon to discuss breast reconstruction. The two of us are side by side on a loveseat in the afternoon light of the waiting room. You would never know we're in a doctor's office. We're unfettered, never stop talking and laughing. When a nurse calls us back, it feels almost like an interruption. *But we were having such a good time,* we might joke.

The nurse leads us to a small room, where she turns on a video. "There you go," she says, and closes the door behind her. The beginning of the film is what I'd call pastel. We witness the joys of reconstruction, its many advantages, hear nice music, see marvelous sunsets lightly smudged by a soft lens. There are loving families, romantic husbands. Then a doctor appears on-screen. Now the colors are crisp, lots of white. The doctor sits behind a very neat desk and explains every possible thing that could go wrong. Then he's gone, and there's another dreamy sunset, more music.

After the film, our same nurse leads us into an exam room, where she takes Brenda's history, instructs her to remove her clothes from the waist up, tie the cotton gown in front. And she leaves. Brenda turns away from me, drops her blouse on the chair, slips into the gown. (I know she's not wearing a bra because bras are still uncomfortable.) By the time she has stepped back up on the table and adjusted the gown beneath her, we hear a knock on the door, and the surgeon enters.

I'm glad his broad back blocks my view. It wouldn't be fair for our usual modesty around each other to fall by the wayside just beside she's in this situation. Oh, yes, he's saying as he examines her, she's an excellent candidate. She'll do well. This will not be difficult. He'll do this, then that—details about the surgery itself, the fine results.

He leaves the room so she can get dressed. He'll return to finalize things, answer questions; then we'll go down the hall to meet with the surgery scheduler. I read a diploma on the wall while Brenda changes into her blouse. After she's buttoned the last button, we both turn at the same time to look each other in the eye. I'm eager to know what she's thinking.

"Why would anybody ever want to do that?" she whispers conspiratorially, shrugging her shoulders the way she does, those shoulders whose shape I know so well.

She's saying the exact words that have been rolling around in my head this entire appointment.

"I agree, Brenda. I totally agree."

She does not have breast reconstruction. She goes on with her life, being the same strong self she has always been. In fact, if you met her—even this soon after her surgery—you would never be able to tell she's had breast cancer. She's a person who knows how to steady herself.

1

Jews don't have coats of arms, but if my family did, it would say, *Sisters Matter*. Adoring your sister is as common a trait in our family as red hair or bowed legs might be in somebody else's.

As rare and expensive as long distance was when I was growing up, Mother and her two sisters called each other more than anyone we knew even *thought* of calling out-of-town relatives. Between calls, Mother would sit at her desk, writing long letters to her older and younger sister, spelling out all the specifics of our lives. Mother would also inquire in detail about her sisters and their families, following up on a niece's toothache or spelling test, the blouse a sister found on sale, wondering if it did indeed go with the skirt she had in mind when she bought it. Back and forth—the breathless letters, phone calls, visits between Mother and her sisters.

Letter written in Yiddish by my grandmother, Bella Bogen, in Denmark, South Carolina, to her sister, Celia Lazin, in Lebanon, Pennsylvania, 1932

But it wasn't just those three sisters who were close. It went back even farther. Mother's mother and *her* sister were also tightly bound. Mother used to tell Brenda and me how, in the early 1900s, our grandmother would take the train—by herself! a woman who barely spoke English! in those days!—all the way from Denmark, South Carolina, to Lebanon, Pennsylvania, to visit her sister. The only mementos I have from my grandmother are eight letters she wrote to Tante Celia in Yiddish—those words like little squiggly designs on a rug, those two sisters like a pair of parentheses, like arms holding something invisible.

Moving into the future, the sister connection will carry through to my identical-twin granddaughters, Lucy and Zoe, who, when they learn to talk, will each call herself and the other "Nay-nay." As though they reside in the same skin. When Lucy looks in the mirror, she'll point to her reflection and proclaim, "Nay-nay!" When Zoe wakes up and sees her sister in the crib across the room, she'll call out, "Nay-nay!"

I talk on the phone with one of them, their voices indistinguishable, and I'll say, "Who is this?"

The answer: "Nay-nay."

They'll begin to say their names when they're two, around the time they learn the word *mine*.

So many sister stories. Brenda and I are part of a design that has existed in our family forever.

When Brenda and I were young-marrieds, Mother treated the two of us, along with her older sister, Emma, to a weekend in North Myrtle Beach. This was before Myrtle Beach turned honky-tonk, when it was still quiet and lovely. We stayed at the Caravelle, an oceanfront motel Mother and her sisters always chose

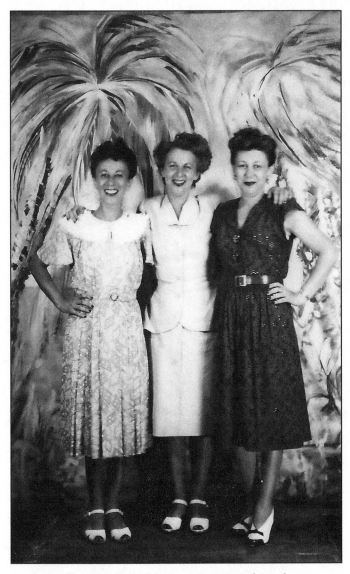

*My mother, Peggy Kurtz, with her sisters, Katie Kahn and
Emma Lavisky, Myrtle Beach, South Carolina, 1947*

because if you got a room on the first floor, you could walk right out your door onto the sand. Aunt Emma and Mother shared a room, Brenda and I a room adjoining theirs.

At breakfast the first morning, in the motel restaurant, Aunt Emma shook salt on her oatmeal, then reached across the table and shook salt on Mother's. Not just a sprinkle. A heavy criss-crossing.

Mother's response, her voice plaintive, good natured, even a little teasing: "But I don't *like* salt on my oatmeal. I like *sugar.*"

The four of us laughed at everything this said about sisters.

2

More sister stories. Breath-thin moments rise back to air:

At five years old, I can always win over my sister by stuffing my whole fist in my mouth. She huddles with neighborhood friends on the sidewalk, engrossed in whatever it is eight-year-olds do. I hang around the outskirts, waiting for a chance to break in. What can I do that they can't? Well, I've been practicing these little tricks. One is saying the alphabet backwards faster than most people can say it forward. But I know that Brenda and her friends will not stay put long enough for me to go from *z* to *a*. Of course, there's this other trick I've perfected. One of Brenda's friends steps back or maybe just turns around briefly, and I quickly slip inside the circle, work my fingers behind my two front teeth, push and grind until my hand disappears all the way up to my bony wrist, and everyone—including my sister—goes, "Goshhh!"

Brenda has me repeat this for other groups. It never fails to astound.

❧

When it's just the two of us, we ballet dance in the front yard, arabesques and piqué turns. We wear the lime and fuchsia crepe-paper dresses that Mattie, the woman who takes care of our household, who's been part of our family since I was three, makes for us. We love the pinked hems, the stiff ruffles like wings. We love Mattie, whose brown hands smell like peaches and can turn anything shimmery.

I follow Brenda through the grass, as though drawn by an invisible cord.

❧

We spend hours in our backyard playhouse. We play school, we play store, we play movie stars. We play and play, humming with summer.

❧

My earliest memory: Six-year-old Brenda is chosen to be flower girl at May Day, a holiday as big in Rock Hill, South Carolina, as Christmas. The day is warm, the sky cloudless. First, the May Court attendants (college students) float down the stone steps of the outdoor amphitheater. Then Brenda, wearing a pink net evening gown trimmed in ribbon, takes her time making the long descent, turning her head from side to side to survey the scenery and drop rose petals from the little white basket on her arm. After a pause, a gap in the procession, comes the queen.

Schoolchildren dance around the Maypole to entertain the court. The attendants, graceful as palms in their pale green dresses, pat their gloved hands together in soft applause. The queen and Brenda, side by side, smile.

Afterward, everyone in the audience pushes down the steps onto the grass to crowd around the queen—and Brenda. "What a smart little girl you are," they say to her. "Those ringlets! Like Shirley Temple!" "You're so pretty!"

At first, she smiles politely, twirling that lock of hair behind her ear she always twirls, and says, "Thank you, thank you." After a while, her response is, "I know, I know."

Mother will tell this story a million times. I love it more with each telling. The appeal is that Brenda is so happy-go-lucky here. Good things are happening. She's smart and pretty and her naturally curly hair is adorable. She's the star, and I'm in the audience. Which suits me just fine.

❧

She's nine, I'm six. She draws a girl with perfect lips. I draw a girl. My lips don't turn out like hers, so I erase, draw again, erase until there's a dark graphite smear on the bottom third of my girl's face, making her look like she needs a shave. Brenda notices my frustration. "Want me to show you how to do lips?" she asks.

When she makes earrings and pins out of seashells from White's Hobby Shop, I make earrings and pins from seashells. We sit at the card table in the den for hours, squeezing the honey-colored glue, sliding the pastel blossoms into place. She changes her design. I change mine. La Petite Beauty Salon places a big order for Brenda's jewelry, sells out, orders more. Brenda objects only a little when Mother asks her if some of my jewelry can be included in the next batch. I would never have thought of such a

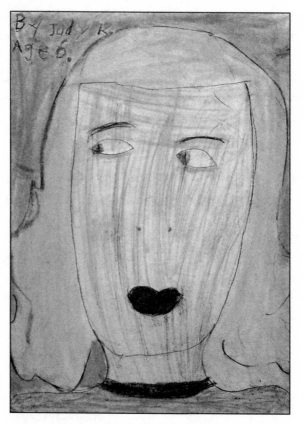

Drawing by me, age 6. Lips by Brenda, age 9.

thing. But Mother says it's what sisters do. BrendaandJudy. We're one long word.

A little older, we publish our own neighborhood newspaper. I write the articles and Brenda illustrates. She's also the marketing director, which means she tells me how far up the street I have to go to sell the papers. I listen carefully. I want to get it exactly right.

❦

I'm afraid of the ball. To cure me, she ties me to a tree in the front yard with our jump rope and throws a basketball at me. Over and over. "See, Judy?" she yells over my sobs. "There's nothing to be scared of. Nothing at all."

❦

I button up my jacket and unlatch the gate in the hedge that separates our backyard from the O'Neals', sprint down their driveway to the sidewalk, aiming for my friend's house, one street and another shortcut away. Up ahead, I see the neighborhood bully in his front yard. He's straight-backed and tall, taller even than Brenda. I can't tell what he's doing. I wave. He looks like he's going to wave back—I think I even see a smile on his hollow-cheeked face—but instead of waving, he hurls a rock in my direction. It hits me square in the forehead, and a spray of blood immediately gums up my vision. The houses on both sides of the street go blurry. My cheeks beat like something electric that's been turned on and forgotten. I spin on my heels, run as fast as I can back home.

As soon as Brenda sees what happened, she bolts out the door. I know where she's going.

Mr. Bully is still in his front yard. Too bad for him. She beats him up so solidly, so thoroughly, that Pernettia, who works for the O'Neals and is outside hanging laundry, hears him screaming and has to run over to pull Brenda off him.

Brenda is just making sure that, where her little sister is concerned, nobody but Brenda gets away with anything.

She was named after Brenda Frazier, a glamorous debutante with whom all of America had fallen in love, who made the cover of *Life* a month before my sister was born, the day after Christmas 1938.

As a child, I memorize that magazine cover—the glorious tangle of brown hair, the little pinched bodice of Brenda Frazier's strapless gown, the way she stares at something out of the camera's range, something I assume only Brendas can see.

My sister has our father's deep-set green eyes and his curly brown hair. She also has his personality and temperament—clear-eyed determination, level-headedness, matter-of-factness, fierce principles, obstinacy. They rely on sensible thinking. The two of them are tall. Their presence: boulder-strong. Everyone tells Brenda, "You are your father to a *T*."

People say Mother and I are just alike. *Sweet* is the word they use to describe us. We rely on feelings. (In fifth grade, I even change my name to Laura Love.) We're both petite, and our facial expressions and gestures mirror each other's, but I'm not beautiful like she is. (Truth is, neither Brenda nor I will grow up to be beautiful.) Heads turn to follow Mother. She could be a double for Elizabeth Taylor, the Elizabeth Taylor in *Giant*, when her makeup is natural and her hair has silvered. Mother's eyes are brown, though, the color of coffee—not lavender. Her face and Elizabeth Taylor's face are both symmetrical, shaped like hearts, crystal-perfect. Like the character in *Giant*, Mother is endearing, open, and attentive to others. She writes thank-you notes in response to thank-you notes. She's the type of person who asks questions, then follow-up questions. She's never just being polite; she's truly interested.

My father is the type who decides whether or not what you want to talk about merits a conversation. He can quite comfortably greet your words with silence. I take that to mean the subjects I care about aren't important enough for him, so I assess what I want to say before I speak, organize sentences in my head before turning them loose. I would never pick boyfriends as a topic, or slumber parties with girlfriends. When I'm older, I'll understand he's just an arm's-length kind of person, that he can be impatient with anyone, and he's strict in his views—there's a right way to do things and a wrong way. He lets you know when you've done it wrong. But oh, the long and expressive letters he writes when something is upsetting your life. Everything will be all right, *you're* all right—more than all right. He's forever proud of you. He lets you know he knows how to love. All this could be said about Brenda as well.

❧

Our father and Brenda are a team. Mother and I are a team.

My brother, eight years older than me, five years older than Brenda, is so unlike the rest of us he could be on loan from another family. He has Mother's brown eyes, and there's something about his chin that's like our father's. But he has his own straight nose and oval face and, even as a young boy, a level of sophistication and wit and remove (and yearning for something bigger and better than our family, than Rock Hill) that makes him seem as though he's speeding toward a different galaxy. If he would just stick around, Brenda and I would gladly crown him king of this galaxy. That's how much the two of us look up to him, lionize him. Well, Brenda looks up to him, so I do, too.

My father's main goal with Donald is to mold him into the perfect son. Make sure he grows up to be ethical and hardworking, traditional enough to want to live in Rock Hill and run The Smart Shop and King's Men's Shop, my father's clothing stores.

All that molding and disciplining—and demand for a life my brother would never choose—feels to Donald like waves of disapproval. Which creates even more distance between him and the rest of our family.

One summer while still in high school, Donald is working at The Smart Shop. His job this Saturday afternoon, the busiest shopping day of the week, is to change the outfits on the mannequins in the front windows. Two of his buddies stop in front of the store. They see him, tap on the glass, and wave. Donald signals them: *Hold on! Wait!* He begins undressing the mannequins one at a time, slowly peeling away their pumps, lifting off their

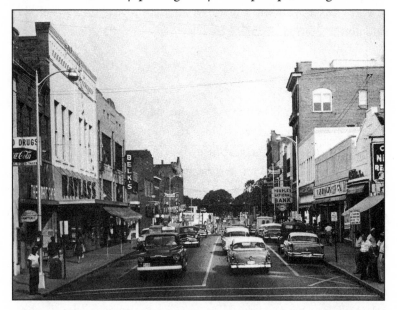

Main Street, Rock Hill, South Carolina, circa 1956. One of my father's stores, The Smart Shop, is on the left.

hats, unbuttoning their dresses, pulling the straps of their nylon slips down their arms. Then, as if the Dixieland jazz that Donald loves were rising all around him, he takes the hand of one of the naked mannequins in his own, circles his arm around her waist, and begins to twirl her. Giddy, he spins her faster and faster. The two of them dance as though they're drunk down to their ankles. Then he chooses another mannequin. Each one waits her turn, smiling, obviously happy for the chance to show that she can keep time to the music. A crowd of shoppers has now joined Donald's pals out front. They laugh and cheer. They even clap.

But then my father hovers in the air above my brother.

Rule number one is, you do not laugh about the store. You certainly don't crack jokes while you're working. This is serious business. Rule number two, you don't waste time while you're working. When you've finished dressing the windows, you check to see if the blouses on the front table need refolding. You make sure the dresses and their hangers are turned the right way.

My father's arms are folded across his chest. For Donald, it's all over.

❧

Brenda and I are having a secret meeting behind the forsythia bush in the backyard.

"So look, Judy," she says, fanning out the girlie magazines.

"In Donald's room?" I whisper with reverence, knowing how grave this is.

"Yep. I found them in his closet," she says. "And look at this."

She holds up a sheet of notebook paper with our brother's artistic handwriting. He's written a story about the TV show *What's My Line?* John Charles Daly, of course, is the moderator who asks the guest to "come in and sign in, please." The guest, a buxom (Donald's exact word) blonde in a tight strapless gown, writes her name on the sign-in board. Dorothy Kilgallen, Arlene Francis, and Bennett Cerf try to guess her vocation. They ask questions that can be answered *yes* or *no*: "Are you salaried? Are you self-employed?" And "Do you deal in a product? A service?" The guest in my brother's episode, it turns out, is a whore (also his word). Neither Brenda nor I allow ourselves to say that word out loud.

Our big decision: what do we do with all this?

We end up doing the only thing we can—bury the magazines and story near the back hedge, deep in the green of the lawn.

The keen electric charge for Brenda: joining our father in helping Donald live a more productive, moral life.

The electric charge for me: colluding with my sister.

❧

When I'm grown and teaching writing workshops, I'll assign this exercise to students: tell the myth surrounding your birth.

Here's mine:

I was born in Rock Hill—unable to swallow. Or maybe it was something about my breathing. I guess it's odd I don't know exactly what was wrong, but that has never been the point of the story.

I was rushed by ambulance from Rock Hill to Columbia, seventy-two miles away, definitely not the closest city. It would've made more sense to take me to Charlotte, only twenty-six miles over the state line. But it was October 20, 1941, a little over a month before Pearl Harbor, and my mother was thirty-one, with a husband and two young children and a newborn near death. She knew that if she could just make it to Columbia, where her two sisters lived, everything would be all right.

Mother wanted to ride with me in the ambulance, but that

was against the rules. The attendant said no; she should follow in the car with my father. The driver said no. The head of the hospital in Rock Hill said no.

She held me, the entire way, on her lap, in the back of the ambulance, on a pink satin pillow.

Days later, I was okay. But Mother never stopped coddling me. Brenda had Daddy. I had Mother. In my eyes, Mother was the prize, the one who was there all the time, the expert at coddling. Which is the point of this story. I've been resting on that satin pillow my whole life.

My sister would probably agree.

Was Brenda coddled by Mother? She would say that Mother *worried* about her, just as she worried about me. But Brenda was so much like Daddy. "Just as stubborn, same temper," Mother would say. "Why, Brenda would sit there in her playpen and throw all her toys out and then scream and scream until I retrieved them for her." Maybe Mother felt that Brenda didn't actually invite coddling.

My parents planned to have only two children. When they had a boy and a girl—"Imagine," my mother said after Donald and Brenda were born, "one of each!"—they decided that would be it. Then I came along. An accident. Not what my parents expected. Not what my sister expected. But Mother turned my birth into something wondrous. Her standard comment about this: "What in the world would we have done without our Judy?"

I just kept arranging myself on that satin pillow, making sure I was as comfortable as could be.

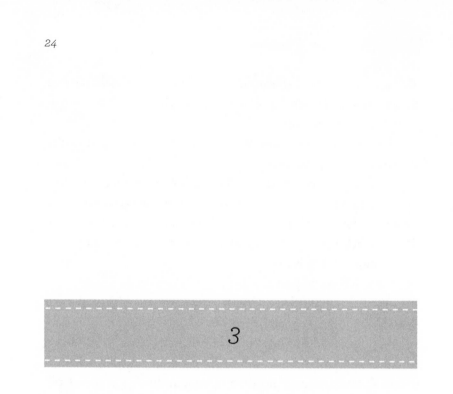

3

It's 1974. I'm thirty-three, married to Henry, with two children—Laurie (five) and Mike (two). My mother-in-law is visiting from Miami, and my mother has driven over from Rock Hill. The three of us are eating turkey sandwiches at my kitchen table in Charlotte. I live in a brick split-level on a street of brick split-levels, all with the same floor plan. The whole neighborhood, in fact, is a looping string of brick split-levels with identical floor plans. Like a toy neighborhood. The front yards are bare except for newly planted willow oak saplings, some straight, some tilting. The day we moved in, I started reading the classifieds again, looking for a house with surprises, a little history and soul. Why did we buy this one? Maybe because the attic fan makes the air smell like the house I grew up in, on Eden Terrace. Maybe because this house was affordable. Maybe because it's only one neighborhood away from—and looks just like—Brenda's.

My mother-in-law, a widow for three years and still so weepy she wears sunglasses indoors, is talking about buying a condominium. When her husband was alive, they lived in an apartment. She still rents but suspects she's throwing her money away. Mother joins her in weighing renting vs. owning.

When Mother comes to the word *condominium*, she stumbles.

"If you buy a con-do-nim-i-um . . . ," she says, not able to unroll the syllables.

I take a big bite of my sandwich. The bread sticks to the roof of my mouth.

Mother is determined. She lights a cigarette, takes a puff. "I mean, con-do-nim-i-um . . ."

She stops and starts again. "A condo . . . ," she says. "Condo . . . Uh, a condo . . ."

Now she's silent, staring out the window at a bush in the backyard as if she's rummaging around in its leaves for the word.

I swallow. "Condominium, Mother."

Why is this bright, articulate woman, who was the only female studying to be a C.P.A. at the University of South Carolina in the 1920s, who kept the books for my father's stores for years, who finishes a crossword puzzle every morning, who loves books, loves writing letters—why is she having such difficulty connecting the vowels and consonants of this ordinary noun?

There are other troubling signs. When we stop by the grocery store, she manages to pay with the right number of dollar bills. But then she dumps all the change from her wallet into her hand —dimes, quarters, pennies loose as copper fish—and holds out her palm for the checkout girl to take what she needs.

I blame everything on her age: she's sixty-five. Of course, our parents are always old to us, even when they're not. How else to explain her confusion, withdrawal, what seems to be depression, the way her feelings get hurt way too easily? Brenda says the problem is that Mother can't cope with losing her beauty. Brenda's assessment irritates me. It makes Mother sound so shallow. As though Brenda is saying, *That sweet person, Peggy Kurtz, whom everyone adores? She's not really so sweet. All she cares about are her looks. I know the real her.*

Brenda's theory denies the most central part of our mother. She *was* beautiful. In fact, she's still beautiful. But if she weren't, it would not matter one bit to her. Her concern has never been herself.

I want to tell Brenda how wrong she is.

I want to tell Brenda her judgment of Mother feels like a judgment of me. That's how gauzy the border is between Mother and me. As though Brenda could also be saying, *That sweet person, Judy? She's not really so sweet. I know the real her.*

4

The next time I'm with my father, I report that Brenda is being impatient with Mother and will he have a talk with her? (I know. I'm being a tattletale.) But he takes Brenda's side, says that he, too, feels impatient at times, which surprises me, considering his legendary devotion to Mother. "Peggy can't unlock the door leading from the garage into the house," he tells me. "She just gives up. She doesn't even try." The first time it happened, she tried to fit the key in the lock, turned it this way and that, kept poking the key into the brass surround as though her fingers didn't belong to her. Finally, she handed him the key and said, "Here, Bennie. You do it."

Mother is certainly not purposely losing her ability to use a key. I tell him maybe she has arthritis. Or she's tired, not getting enough sleep. Maybe she has a lot on her mind.

Brenda, Daddy, and I have three distinct interpretations of what we're seeing, all reflecting our individual personalities and our differing relationships with Mother. But we have one thing in common: none of us wants to admit how sick she is.

One night, my father, Henry, and I are at Brenda and Chuck's for dinner. Mother is in Columbia, visiting her sisters. Before we get to the table, before we even take off our coats—in the front hall, under that merciless light—we start comparing notes. *Do you realize Mother can no longer look up numbers in the phone book? Have you noticed she now wears only pants with elastic waists, no buttons or zippers, easy to get on and off? How long has it been since she's written a letter?* The words are like matches striking.

5

Our father takes Mother to a neurologist in Charlotte. Days later, a receptionist calls Brenda with the diagnosis. The doctor doesn't call. His nurse doesn't call. His receptionist calls. And whom does she call? Not the patient. Not the patient's husband. The patient's daughter (who then, of course, calls me). Did the doctor not want to spring for a long-distance call from his office in Charlotte, North Carolina, to my parents in Rock Hill, South Carolina? Did he think the news was so bleak it didn't warrant a face-to-face meeting with my parents? *Here's the problem. There's nothing we can do about it. You're on your own, folks.*

Of course, Brenda and I don't realize it's easier to focus on the delivery of the news than the news itself. We're too young, too inexperienced, to know we're fixating on one small piece that will ultimately be beside the point, just so we can avoid burrowing down through grief.

Now we're focusing—and disagreeing—on how the news will be delivered to our parents.

Brenda thinks we should tell our father first and let him decide how, when—whether—to tell Mother. I want to tell them
together. After all, it's her illness. Doesn't she deserve to know?
And doesn't she deserve to know at the same time everyone else
knows?

I tell Brenda what I think. She tells me what she thinks—
again.

The final decision: Brenda will call our father, arrange for the
two of us to meet him at Shoney's in the Rock Hill Mall, where
his stores are now, and she and I will tell him in person. Without
Mother.

Normally, I don't even notice I'm letting Brenda talk me into
something. What's new here is that I actually voice disagreement
with her. I speak up! But it's such risky behavior (she could get
angry, she probably knows best anyway) that I quickly go silent,
slip into her way of thinking as easily as I used to slip under the
parrot-colored quilt on my childhood bed, next to hers.

Brenda pushes open the doors of Shoney's and walks ahead.
I hold back, wait for my eyes to adjust to the dimness, spot our
father alone in a booth near the back. He's in his shirtsleeves. His
brown tweed jacket is folded long, then short, beside him, and he
already has his iced tea. He waves a small wave. It's late afternoon,
so the place is quiet, except for one table of waitresses near the
front and their world-weary chatter.

My father slides out of the booth to give each of us a kiss.
He's cheery. So cheery, in fact, grinning his lopsided grin, that
for a minute I can pretend we're here to plan a glittery surprise
birthday party for Mother. We'll set up tables in my empty living
room, freeze casseroles ahead. I'll buy a new outfit.

But no. Brenda gets right down to business. We're still posi-
tioning ourselves in the booth, she and I on one side, our father

across, when she begins telling about the phone call from the doctor's office.

I glance from our father to Brenda, one a shadow of the other. Their faces are roundish, nicely shaped, not long and thin like mine. I could sketch the profile they share, the way their foreheads slope outward and their noses turn up slightly. My father is a slim five-eleven. Brenda, a just-as-slim five-eight. Whenever I stand next to her, I'm struck by how tall she is. I'm under five-three. When we're walking together, I can barely keep up with her long strides.

"The news about Mother isn't good, Daddy. It's Alzheimer's disease. Mother has early-onset dementia." Brenda's words are close together and match her breaths. I can tell she's trying to keep from crying. Her glasses are a little crooked, but she doesn't bother straightening them. "There's nothing they can do for her, so we have to prepare ourselves. It's a neurological disorder that'll only get worse."

This is 1975. People know about senility but not Alzheimer's disease. Rita Hayworth has just been diagnosed with Alzheimer's. Her daughter, Princess Yasmin Aga Khan, is in magazines and newspapers everywhere, trying to raise public awareness of the disease. You can't miss the anguish in her face, the look that says, *Somebody, do something. This can't be happening to my mother. She's too beautiful. Too important.*

"Mother will have more and more trouble remembering things," Brenda is saying. None of us is taking a menu from the clip on the paper-napkin holder. I look at my father but can't read his face. "She'll get lost, even in familiar surroundings. Soon she won't be able to recognize her own family. And she'll become violent."

I fiddle with an earring, try to decide if I should contradict my sister. Decide. "Well, she *might* become violent."

Brenda contradicts *me*. "She *will* become violent." And for backup: "That is what the lady from the doctor's office said."

And because the lady called Brenda, does that make Brenda captain of this illness?

"I understand," I say, "that people who have Alzheimer's disease lose their memory. What I have a hard time believing is that every single person with Alzheimer's becomes violent."

"Well, that is what I was told."

"But by a receptionist!"

"Judy." How does she manage to get across so much just by saying my name?

In my wildest dreams, I cannot imagine Mother being violent. What does *violent* even mean? Stomping her feet in a fit of temper? Bullying someone? Hitting? It's not going to happen. I'd bet my life.

Again, Brenda's assertion feels like a judgment of Mother. How can she be so sure Mother will become violent? Is she suggesting this is something she's seen in Mother all along?

I'm jumping to conclusions, but I can't help it.

A waitress comes over and asks if we've decided what we want. Her hair is brown and unruly. A waitress should not have unruly hair. Right now, I don't want unruly anything.

"Water for me," Brenda says.

"I'll have water, too, please," I say.

My father just sits there, fingering his jaw. After a few seconds, he stirs his tea, then tastes it. The waitress moves away, pushing in on the sides of her hair, as if that'll do any good.

"They call this sweet tea?" he says to no one. The glass is sweating in his hand. "Mattie needs to come down here and give somebody lessons."

He puts down the tea and closes his eyes. He doesn't say another word. Brenda and I sit and wait. His palms are flat on the table.

Finally, eyes still closed, he says, "Well, let's see what the Mayo Clinic has to say."

So. He's not accepting the diagnosis. Good. If he doesn't buy it, none of us has to. We can unsee the troubling signs we've been seeing. What if we *are* making a big deal out of nothing? There are days when Mother seems fine. On the drive over to meet our father, I even said to Brenda, "I know lots of older women who are a little forgetful, and nobody is saying *they* have Alzheimer's."

Brenda kept her hands locked on the steering wheel. All she said was, "Judy."

This scene in Shoney's will find its way, along with the biopsies and Brenda's breast cancer, into my first novel, *The Slow Way Back*. While I'm working on the manuscript, I won't be able to imagine ever changing course and writing about my sister and me directly—head on—in a memoir. The closest I can come at this point is to deal with us obliquely, in fiction. Which means I work through the material at a distance, not up close. Put us in an invented story. Two sisters who are sort of made up, sort of not, doing some made-up, some not-made-up, things.

6

In our family, the Mayo Clinic in Rochester, Minnesota, is the final word on health. My parents flew there over the years with Mother's two sisters and their husbands just to get checked out, as though it were some kind of luxury spa with lounge chairs beside a pool. Their first time, everyone but Mother got a "clean bill of health." It turned out she needed thyroid surgery. I remember Mother and my aunts laughing about this, turning it into another family story: Peggy was the only one who hadn't gone with a specific ailment, who'd been feeling fine, and she was the one who ended up needing an operation. Still, whatever the doctors at Mayo said was true; you could count on it.

This time, my parents fly to Mayo in the middle of winter—January—alone.

When they return, Henry and I pick them up at the Charlotte airport and drive them home to Rock Hill. Henry left his office early today (he's an optometrist) so he can be with me when I hear the diagnosis. That's the type of husband he is. If it's an icy morning, he'll scrape my car windows before leaving for work. If one of us travels without the other, we both leave love notes— taped to the bathroom mirror or the egg carton in the fridge, tucked into a shoe in the traveler's suitcase. We've been doing this all our married life. Our marriage isn't perfect—he yells when he's angry, I'm always trying to make him over—but we're solid.

My parents tell us everything *but* the diagnosis. They talk about the underground tunnel from their hotel to the hospital, how they never ventured outside because the city was frozen hard. Mother asks about Laurie and Mike, about Brenda and Chuck and their boys—David, Brian, Scott, and Danny. What have we heard from Donald? (He and his wife, Mara, and their daughter, Sasha, live in New York City.) How is Mattie? It isn't until we've brought in the suitcases and are seated around the breakfast-room table, eating the caramel cake Mattie left on the counter with a welcome-home note, that my parents tell the real news of the trip.

First, the different tests—many more than the neurologist in Charlotte ran. Then, this morning, just before they left, how the doctor sat across from them in his private office and delivered the results. They both heard the diagnosis: Alzheimer's disease. And they both heard the prognosis.

Wait a minute, I want to say. *Hold everything!* I hate that Mother knows. How can she possibly cope with the knowledge that the promise of her is gone? But then, what *do* I want? It wasn't okay that the doctor in Charlotte did not tell my mother. It wasn't okay that Brenda and I didn't tell her. And now it's not okay that the doctor at Mayo did tell her. What is okay?

Later that evening, my father and Henry watch the news in

the living room. I hunch on the low stool in Mother's closet, my face tilted up toward her as she steps out of her wool pants. When she twists to pull off her long-sleeved slipover sweater, I stand to help. She raises both arms like a child. They hang in the air. I pull off her sweater and fold it away on the shelf. She holds on to my shoulder while I take her shoes, one at a time. She's tired, I can tell. So tired. She rolls off her pantyhose, her panties, and turns so I can unhook her bra. In a gesture of respect—a nod toward decorum—I glance away at the corner, where wall meets wall.

When I look back, she's holding her nylon nightgown. I accordion it up, hold it over her head, and let it down over her shoulders, the full length of her body. She lowers her chin, and I see that she's crying quietly. No sound. Only the tears, which make her cheeks wet and pearly. I hand her a Kleenex from the decorative wooden box on her dressing table.

She dabs her eyes. "The first thing I said to the doctor at Mayo was, 'How in the world am I going to tell my daughters?'"

Which is unsettling and reassuring. Both.

Unsettling, because it means she understands what this diagnosis means. She has always put all her eggs in one basket: communication. She believes nothing is so tough that we can't discuss it. In fact, talking about difficult things is what gets us to the other side. But this news is *so* tough, *so* difficult, she didn't know how she could possibly tell us. It's clear she understands exactly what lies ahead.

At the same time, her response is reassuring. For now, at least, my mother is still very much herself. Her main concern: How will she protect her daughters? How can she comfort us, guard us, keep us safe?

7

Mother and I are elbow to elbow on the sofa in her living room. Her small, dangly mother-of-pearl earrings twist as she turns her face toward Brenda and me. Brenda is to my left, in Daddy's deep brown chair, her long legs stretched across the ottoman. This is weeks after the Mayo diagnosis.

"Don't you just love this house? Aren't we lucky to be here?" Mother says cheerily. She begins every conversation that takes place on Pinewood Lane this way, opening both arms to take in the margins of the room, every bookshelf and doorknob.

When I was fourteen, she and my father announced to Donald, Brenda, and me that they'd bought property in Country Club Estates, on the outskirts of town, where they would build a smaller house, a brick ranch. They'd sell the two-story white clapboard house with grey shutters on Eden Terrace, minutes from school and every one of my friends, the only home I'd ever known.

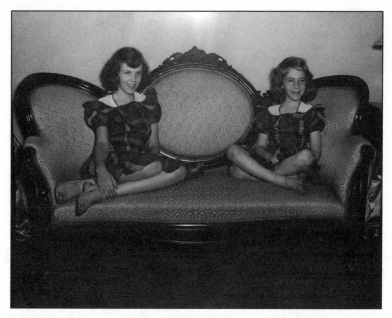

With Brenda in the living room of the house on Eden Terrace, 1949

Brenda, a year away from graduating high school and always interested in houses and design, was immediately spinning with ideas for paint colors, carpeting, kitchen counters. Donald was in his last year at the University of North Carolina, about to achieve the independence he'd always craved. Even when he was younger, he would not have had an attachment to the house. A ninth-grader, I buried my face in my hands. Made sure everyone *saw* that I was burying my face in my hands.

How could we just pack up and leave?

Why would we want to leave our knotty-pine den with the floor-to-ceiling bookshelves, the family photographs covering the wall surrounding the mantel, the double window sills and their row of African violets? Brenda's and my desks, facing opposite corners?

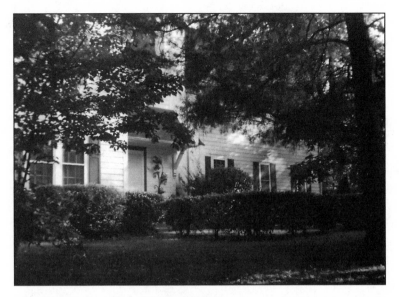

842 Eden Terrace, Rock Hill, South Carolina

Our living room—its Victorian sofa, damask draperies, baby grand.

The breakfast room with the built-in painted cupboards.

Our tiny screened porch with the clothes dryer and the wooden crate of Cokes on top.

The swimming pool in the backyard (built three years earlier, when Rock Hill Concrete Company wanted to break into the pool business and we were happy to be part of their experiment), the little cabana (once Brenda's and my playhouse) with the stacks of beach towels and bathing suits for any guests who forgot theirs. Days, Brenda and I would float on rafts, the straps of our suits pulled off our shoulders for a more even tan, a radio balanced in our open upstairs bedroom window, blaring music. Nights, the two of us ducked underwater when bats dove down for a sip.

Brenda's and my room. Our twin beds facing the fireplace, our matching quilts. Our square little closets with the faceted glass doorknobs.

Why would we ever want to leave Eden Terrace?

Brenda said I was being silly. Mother said she understood how I felt—and talked my father into selling the property they'd just bought. They would postpone moving till after I'd left home for good.

Eight years later, after I'd graduated from college, they bought a different lot, one with a sloping front yard and a great bonus for my father: it backed up to the thirteenth hole on the golf course, which meant he could walk out the back door after dinner and hit shots up and down the fairway till dark. Watching from the window, you could tell by the way he held that long, lanky body of his that he was humming to himself.

Mother's take on the way things turn out is always how lucky we are. As though our lives were hanging in the balance and we miraculously caught hold and were saved. She's that way over this house. *The first lot was so wrong! Thank goodness we didn't build on that one!* She can be the same way over a pair of shoes for Brenda or me. *Aren't we lucky you found those flats? We could've looked forever and not found any so perfect!*

I kick off my shoes and pull my legs up under me. Mother reaches for the cigarette box on the glass coffee table, lights up, blows smoke out the side of her mouth, away from Brenda and me.

"Something very frightening happened, girls." Her eyes are suddenly dark with confusion. She's obviously off the subject of the house and onto something else. "Yesterday, I went to the drugstore and couldn't find my way home. The drugstore! Right on Cherry Road! I was driving around and around and had no idea where I was. After a long time, I found myself all the way out at Rock Hill Feed and Supply. How could I not know my way around Rock Hill? It felt like a circuit had been broken in my brain."

"Oh, Mother," is all I can think to say.

Brenda says, "Maybe there's some kind of medication that would help. I think Daddy should get in touch with the doctor at Mayo."

"Well, let's see if it happens again," Mother says.

"That makes sense," I say. "Let's just wait."

Carefully, Mother places her half-smoked cigarette (for years, her way of cutting back) in the little brass ring in the ashtray, one of those gadgets she's always ordering from catalogs. This one puts out the fire without letting smoke rise in the room.

Immediately, Brenda reports all this to our father. He calls the doctor at Mayo, who reminds him there's nothing he can prescribe for Alzheimer's.

The disease advances. Mother is still driving, but Brenda and I both see that even when she's making her way from one side of the living room to the other, she bumps the legs of tables and chairs. Imagine how she steers a car.

The big question: who's going to take away her keys? Brenda says our father should do it. I know in my heart she's right, but for some reason, I say no, not him, I'm the one who should do it.

Am I going up against Brenda just to go up against Brenda? Mother shows more and more signs of illness, and I grow more and more determined to show a side of myself none of us knows?

It turns out Mother takes matters into her own hands. After all, she's the mother who wrote us excuses from school if we were tired, who told us not to work so hard, that Bs were just as good as As.

As if she can still spare me, before I have a chance to even broach the subject—at the Saluda Road intersection, two blocks from the house—she runs a stop sign and hits another car. Neither she nor the other driver is hurt. I don't have to say a word. She doesn't get behind the wheel again.

Mother's friends are dropping away. Very few phone calls or visits or invitations. I understand it's not easy to be around her now; she's slower, quieter, dull. What I don't understand is when one of her friends—or Brenda—sees the symptoms of Alzheimer's as personality traits she's always had. "Well, you know how she can be forgetful" is one comment. Mother was *never* forgetful. Or: "She's always been a little depressed." Mother was *known* for her buoyancy. I want to say, *This is not our mother! Don't you see? Just because the sky changes color, can't you remember when it was blue?*

8

Back in 1971 (before Mother's Alzheimer's), my father had co-lon cancer, surgery, no chemo or radiation necessary. Future rosy.

Now, five years later, 1976, he's diagnosed with lung cancer. Surgery again. We're relieved the new tumor is small and the doctor is able to get it all. His prognosis, the doctor says, is excellent.

Weeks pass. He has a follow-up exam. Things don't look so hopeful after all. It's now in his bones.

He's weak from the lung surgery and even weaker from the bone cancer that's ambushing his body. Too weak to think of going to the Mayo Clinic. My brother pleads with him to come to Memorial Sloan-Kettering. Donald even makes an appointment for him with a doctor who's on the cover of *New York* magazine's "Best Doctors in New York City" issue, who also happens to be Nelson Rockefeller's doctor. (Donald is trying so hard. I have a feeling he's not only hoping to help Daddy but also wants to show him how high powered and well connected he is.) Our father says no. He can't manage a plane trip and doesn't want to leave Mother.

Eventually, though, he says yes to Donald, which is significant for three reasons: First, we'll hear a definitive prognosis from cancer specialists—this is before there are oncologists in smaller cities. Second, he's allowing himself to be taken care of, which is not something he normally would be willing to do. Third and most important, he's taking Donald's advice—unexpected acknowledgment that maybe his son *is* someone he can rely on.

Naturally, Brenda flies to New York with our father and I stay home to look after Mother. This is decided without our even having to discuss it.

Mattie will be at the house during the day to cook and take care of Mother, and the night aide my father hired for the time he's away will come in for her shift. Mornings, I'll drive over to Rock Hill to help Mattie, keep Mother company, shop, run errands. I can be back in Charlotte in time to get my work done (I have a freelance advertising copywriting business) and pick up Laurie and Mike from school.

It's March, and just as I arrive the first day, an ice storm comes skidding in, which makes Highway 21 unnavigable and every town within a hundred-mile radius ice-locked. Not only is it impossible for me to drive home, the aide can't get to the house.

Of course, Mattie is here; she would never *not* come. She lives ten minutes away, rides with the woman who works for the family next door.

Mattie has been with us since 1944, when she was twenty-six. In the early years, she lived with us on Eden Terrace. In fact, she and I shared a room, a double bed. I adored her soft and boundless bosom, her soft and boundless everything. When my parents added a master bedroom upstairs and a living room below,

Brenda and I moved into our parents' old bedroom and Mattie got her own room. She was married then, but working for us meant she did not live with her husband. I never heard Mattie's views on this; it's not something she would have discussed. But I can remember feeling sad for her, for this arrangement—until, on one of her nights off, her husband came to pick her up. When my father opened the front door, Jay was so drunk he practically fell into the entrance hall. He was bellowing crazy things, cursing Mattie. Brenda and I huddled together on the upstairs landing, listening, our heads poking through the wooden slats of the banister. Why was he so mad at Mattie? We couldn't make out his words. "Go on home now, Jay," we heard our father say as he gently guided Jay back out the door. The next day, Mattie found out that Jay had a gun the night before and was going to shoot her. My father helped her take out a restraining order, and that was the last any of us heard of Jay. I don't think they ever divorced, but the marriage was over. Five or six years later, she was able to buy a small wood-frame house for herself. Not long after she moved in, her house burned down. My parents then built her a three-bedroom brick house in a neighborhood close to theirs, and she has lived there ever since.

For now, for however long it takes the ice to melt, my mother, Mattie, and I will be here.

Mother paces. Her stooped shoulders and jutting chin propel her in a lurching way—from the windows overlooking the golf course, through the living room, to the front door. Stop, wheel, back again. Her speech is hesitant; she can manage only one or two broken sentences at a time. She says things over and over. I can tell she feels lost without my father. Every few minutes, another anxious question: "When is Bennie coming home? Where'd he go?" I remind her that he's in the hospital in New York, that Brenda and Donald are with him. And then I remind her again.

The days are long. She can't read, not even a magazine or a newspaper. She can't sit long enough to watch TV. She still smokes,
but I have to light her cigarettes and watch to be sure she doesn't
leave one burning. Watching, in fact, is about all I can do. Watch
for fire. Watch for a break in the weather. Watch the disintegra-
tion of my mother.

I try to come up with ideas to fill the hours. Mother, Mattie,
and I organize the linen closet, find a bedspread that's perfect for
the guest room in Mattie's house. "Aren't we lucky we found it?"
Mother says a dozen times. Now I'm beginning to feel impatient.
I had no idea I'd be staying this long. I want to go home to my
husband and children.

"Is there anything here *you* need?" she asks in a wistful voice.
We're in the kitchen. Mattie is in the laundry room, folding
clothes. I've just poured Cokes for us, and I'm searching the cabi-
nets for a snack, something crunchy. Fritos? A Snickers bar?

"No. Thanks. I really don't need anything," I answer.

"Surely, there's something."

"No, there's really nothing here I need."

Too late, I realize *her* need is the subject of our conversation.

Her face tightens and she says, "Look around. I really want . . . to
give you a present."

Now I'm feeling guilty—why won't I just pick something?—
but I can't begin to think what in the house I might want.
Things are my last concern right now. How I'm going to get to
the grocery store to buy food for our supper is what concerns me.
How long am I going to have to stay here? How is Henry manag-
ing with the children? What about my work?

I put the kettle on. I'm not sure why. My glass of Coca-Cola
is right here.

"How about this?" she offers, taking the majolica vase from
the center of the breakfast-room table and turning it slowly in her

hands, as though she works in an antique store and is pointing out the vase's features—the glassy lilac-pink flower on the chalk-like, pebbly surface. She tilts the vase to show me its glassy lilac-pink throat.

"Okay. I'd love to have that." I turn the water off before it boils. I don't say that I know the vase well, that she doesn't need to show it to me in such detail, that we've had it for as long as I can remember.

"Good." She laughs gaily, the way she used to. "Real good." She laughs again. It's the laugh of a mother who can still do for her child.

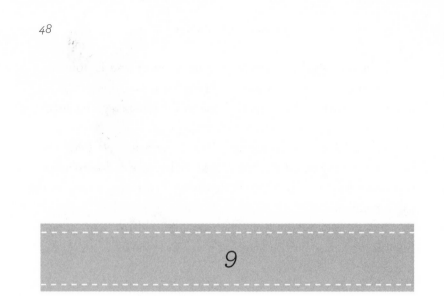

9

I stay with Mother three nights. Finally, the ice melts enough for me to drive home to Charlotte. Mattie will sleep at the house until the aide returns.

At home, I take steamy baths that last half the morning. I can't get enough of cuddling with Laurie and Mike. Henry and I talk into the night. I crawl back into bed after lunch. Overdue work projects collect on my desk. My mother-in-law, who moved from Miami to Charlotte, invites me over for a bowl of her home-made chicken and rice soup. It feels so good to have someone take care of me that I start crying when I try to thank her. I understand why my father is still working. Mother's life is a life full of nothing. And it's exhausting to witness.

I don't stay home long. I'm dying to join Brenda and our father in New York. At home, Mother's illness is a wallop, but maybe in New York the outlook will be brighter.

When I arrive at Memorial Sloan-Kettering, our father is

sleeping. Brenda is sitting on the foot of his bed, Donald in a chair across the room. Brenda and I have a lot to catch up on. Daddy is hard-of-hearing in his right ear and he's lying on his left side, so we can talk without waking him. Our hands make a fluttery pattern—our fingers fold and open—as I report on Mother and she reports on our father. Our new caregiver roles make us feel important.

"The doctor is really nice," she says. "He'll probably end up doing more surgery or maybe start some kind of treatment. Anyway, when the test results are in, he'll come talk to us."

Donald adds, "He sounded optimistic."

Before I flew to New York, Brenda told me during a phone conversation that this hospital stay has been a good thing for Daddy and Donald. Donald has spent long hours with him. And for the first time, Daddy has taken an interest in Donald's ad agency. In the past, our father's opinion was that advertising is not a real business. When Donald moved to New York and started working at Benton & Bowles Advertising, our father came to the city on a business trip for his stores. Before dinner one evening, he met Donald at his office, in that grand building at 666 Fifth Avenue. As Donald showed him around—the creative department (with all the kooky stuff tacked to the walls), account management (Donald's area: the heavy drapes, cushy chairs)— our father whispered, half kidding, half something else, "What kind of a business is this? I don't see a single cash register!"

And then the doctor enters my father's room. He walks in boldly, but not in a rush. He looks at each of us. I'm leaning against the wall next to Brenda, still wearing my heavy coat and holding my purse. My suitcase is on the floor beside me. I introduce myself.

Our father opens his eyes and smiles at me. I lean over to kiss his cheek. Donald gives the doctor his chair, and the doctor slides across the floor close to our father. His words are matter-of-fact and sure. He has the test results, he says. The tumor that was recently discovered in the lung was not the primary tumor and should not have been removed. The primary tumor is in the colon, which means this is a recurrence of that cancer. And it has metastasized. If the doctors in Charlotte had been more thorough in their testing (hesitation here—obvious he doesn't want to point a finger), the primary tumor would have been located and removed, and the others (actually, more than one in the lung) would more than likely shrink on their own or through treatment. If that were the case, my father would be facing a better prognosis. As it is, there's nothing more the doctors can do for him. He can have radiation in Charlotte to alleviate the pain from the bone cancer. He'll be discharged from Sloan-Kettering tomorrow.

Okay. Both of our parents are going to die. And we know *how* they'll die. Mother is sixty-seven. Daddy, sixty-eight.

The doctor looks at his hands, then at our father. He touches our father's shoulder, bare because his gown is twisted. "Do you have any questions, Mr. Kurtz?"

"No," our father says. "I just thank you for all you've done."

"Anyone? Questions?"

"No," Donald says.

"No questions," Brenda says.

"No. No questions," I say.

I do have a question, but I can't ask it, not in front of our father. Brenda and Donald can't either. *How much time does he have?*

The doctor leaves, and the four of us are alone. Our father refolds the hem of the sheet over the waffled blanket and smoothes out the wrinkles. He kicks the covers off his feet. We all know he likes those narrow, size-twelve feet out, in the cool air. Brenda and I both reach over to pat a foot. Her hand lingers. It's shaking a little.

Even though our father will be discharged tomorrow morning, Donald has to jump through hoops at the hospital to get permission to take him out for dinner tonight. But my brother is determined. After refusals from the nurse and nursing supervisor, he finally gets an okay from the attending physician. Donald hires a car and driver to take the four of us to the Coach House Restaurant on Waverly Place in the Village, a fitting choice because it has the atmosphere of a bygone way of life, much like the privileged South of the 1940s and 1950s—elderly and elegant black waiters taking care of every little request, fine tablecloths and napkins, limited menu of chicken pie, prime rib cooked as rare or well done as you like, lamb chops, pecan pie. Bountiful portions. I'm embarrassed to say it feels like home. How pampered (for us) and patronizing (for the waiters) it all is. Still, the polite murmurings and tinkle of china and crystal allow me to pretend that, for us as a family, nothing has changed. In this hushed and snug place, we're as far from medical charts, technology, and bad outcomes as we can be.

It's one of those evenings when nerve endings feel closer than normal to the surface of the skin, in the way that, in the midst of great sadness, life can slow and spirits soar. We drink wine and eat more than we should and laugh and tell our glad-to-be-part-of-this-family stories. You would never know our father is sick. He tells more stories than anyone. The one we all know but don't mind hearing again: When he and Mother met at the Key Club dance in 1930, when she was Miss Key Club (and Miss Denmark and runner-up to Miss South Carolina), how he arrived at the dance late, cut in on her, told her she was just the type of girl

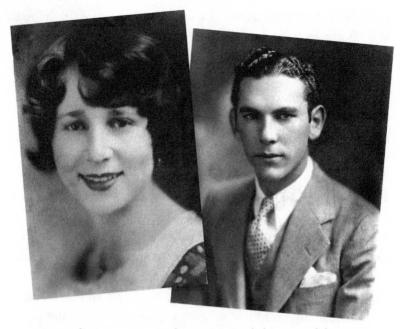

Our mother's engagement photo, 1931. Our father, around the same time.

he detested, Miss Beautiful, everybody's sweetheart, how she told him he was just the type of boy she detested, drunk, bottle under the table. On and on. They met again months later. Fell in love. Married January 3, 1932, the day after the banks closed.

None of us notices that the restaurant has emptied until Donald jokes, "We've been sitting here so long, my shoes have gone out of style!" Which brings the biggest laugh of the evening. I love when our father laughs that laugh where he raises his shoulders almost up to his ears.

We thank the waiters, apologize for keeping them so late, help each other into our coats and out to the car. The night has gotten colder. Wind heaves down and stings our faces. People pass us on the sidewalk, moving in and out of the shadows. Brenda pulls our father's wool scarf up around his neck, and the driver swings open the rear door. He takes my father's elbow and guides him inside. He steers Brenda around to the other side. I settle in on my father's right, Brenda his left. Donald slides in front with the driver. We're still telling stories and laughing.

As we pull away from the curb, I take a quick look back. For a second, the lanterns flanking the doors of the restaurant appear bright enough to light up the whole city.

10

Once Brenda is home, she jumps right into such a busy schedule, it seems she has already accepted our father's fate. In her pragmatic, no-nonsense, definite way, she's simply doing what *he* has always done. One of his pet sayings: "If you're going to do business, you have to do it in today's market." He does not live in the past. He does not put up with regrets. If a shipment of blouses arrives later than promised, if the Christmas season is a little slow, you just deal with it. *If this is the way it is, my job is to adjust.*

I decide *my* job is to call our father's doctor in Charlotte (whom I know, but not well) to tell him what the doctor at Memorial Sloan-Kettering said. The real reason for my call: I want him to admit his mistake.

Of course, it's not like me to speak up. I'm thirty-five and have never been one to challenge people in authority. But it feels as though the unfairness of life has smacked me head-on. My safe and protected childhood amounted to a promise. "Cast your bread upon the waters," Mother used to say, which I took to mean that if I were *sweet*, if I did the right thing, if I were polite enough, the pretty surface of my entitlement would never be shattered.

I thought I was special. An exception to the rule.

I was not prepared for happenstance.

I want to hold someone accountable.

I grip the phone. If I ease up even a little, it could slip out of my hand. The doctor is telling me they did a particular type of surgery because of such-and-such and it was the right thing to do because of such-and-such and there are grey areas in medicine and all in all, big picture, my father's course of treatment was correct. I stare at the light fixture above my kitchen table and press him. I'm not interested in a lawsuit, I assure him, or even an apology; I just want the truth. I flick on the light. Reflections fly off like bits of stone.

The doctor is masterful at defending his actions. "Wait, wait," I say, but he interrupts me to defend even more. Now he's using such esoteric language, he could be speaking Portuguese.

I can't stand it any longer. I raise my voice: "Tell the truth! You missed it! And it did not have to be this way!"

Whatever was coiled inside me like a fist is *un*coiling. "Because of your error in judgment"—now I'm yelling and stomping my foot on every word—"my father is going to die sooner than he should!"

This is the first whiff of what Henry and I will later jokingly call my "hospital personality." It will manifest itself whenever someone close is seriously ill. Instead of accepting how little control I have, I'll double up on my vigilance. I'll keep a watchful and suspicious eye, ask doctors and nurses a million questions. I'll honestly believe—during my most extreme moments—that if

I'm alert, if nothing escapes my attention, if I check behind every doctor and nurse and weigh every decision, I can avert a catastrophe, swoop in and save my loved one.

I'm standing in my kitchen with the brown- and blue-flowered wallpaper. I'm suddenly aware that Laurie (eight) and Mike (five) are at my side—how long have they been here?—looking for something in my face that will explain why I'm yelling. I feel their little hands around my legs, as though they're holding me down, trying to put a stop to this swift unwinding. I know it's time to start dinner, but all I can do is try to keep this phone conversation going.

"Admit it!" I'm screaming at the top of my voice. "Admit it!"

"Judy, Judy, calm down," the doctor says. Then he takes a long pause. And quietly and quickly, as if *quiet* and *quick* translate into *not incriminating,* he says, "Okay. We may have made a mistake."

"Thank you," I say, soft-voiced again, and hang up. I wipe my hand—the one that held the phone—on the side seam of my jeans and turn toward the refrigerator and the ground chuck and sesame-seed buns that will be our dinner. I'm too tired to open a can of baked beans to go with the hamburgers. Too worn out to think of slicing an onion and a tomato.

Later, when I tell Brenda what I did, she just looks at me. She doesn't say a word. I know what she's thinking. She doesn't like my new hospital personality.

11

I pick up Brenda and we drive to Rock Hill. It's early 1979. Our plan is to spend the morning with Mother. Then the three of us will meet Daddy for lunch at Shoney's, spend the afternoon shopping together in his store.

When we arrive at the house, Mattie tells us that last night was not good for our parents. "Miss Peggy's been doing some peculiar things in the middle of the night," Mattie says.

"Like what?" we ask.

"Like getting up and wrapping the alarm clock in a towel and throwing it in the trash can. Like crawling all over the covers and screaming, 'Get me out of this box!' Like wandering around the house, not knowing nothing."

Last night, my father woke to find the other side of the bed empty. He pulled himself up, couldn't find Mother anywhere, saw the front door ajar, stepped out into the pitch dark. She was running barefoot, in the middle of the street, down the hill toward the tall weeds surrounding the lake.

Our new plan for today: Mother will stay home and nap. Neither Brenda nor I feels like shopping now. We'll just meet our father at Shoney's, then head back to Charlotte.

At lunch, the conversation, of course, centers on Mother, what's next, "how this thing will go," to use my father's words. But then we launch into chitchat—his golf game, the grandchildren—as though the world rolled over and is normal again. It's a good thing. We all need a breather.

Brenda is telling about the majolica she has started collecting, how she finds pitchers, plates, and vases at flea markets for next to nothing. She collects the glazed nineteenth-century earthenware because she likes the design, the deep colors. Whether it ever becomes valuable (it will) is not as important to her.

She asks if she can have the small majolica vase that sits on my kitchen table, the one Mother gave me.

I see the expectation in my sister's face. In *my* face, I'm sure she and my father see reluctance. I'm thinking about the day Mother put it in my hands. How many years had it sat in the center of the breakfast-room table in the house on Pinewood Lane and, before that, on Eden Terrace?

Before I can turn to my sister and stammer an answer, my father says, "Brenda, you have the right to ask. And Judy, you have the right to say no."

"Well, I really would like to keep it," I say, looking from my father to Brenda.

"Okay," she says. "That's okay." Not a shadow crosses her face.

This flash thought crosses my mind: *If he could just stay alive, if Mother could stay lucid—both parents alive and well—not only would Brenda and I be looked after, our relationship would be looked after.*

12

Our daughter, Laurie, is almost ten and has never spent a full night away from home. "I think I can make it this time," she'll say as she stuffs her Big Bird pajamas into an overnight bag. But around eleven o'clock, we get the soggy phone call saying she misses her bed and wants to come home. Then the quiet ride home and her falling asleep with her sad little head on Henry's or my shoulder. Then the next try.

One day, she informs us she wants to attend Camp Seafarer this summer, a five-week camp on the coast in Arapahoe, North Carolina. Five weeks? For a child who has never spent a full night away? Plus, Arapahoe is about as far as you can travel from Charlotte and still be in North Carolina—a six-and-a-half-hour drive. But Henry and I sense that she knows what's best for herself, and if this is what she wants, we'll try to make it happen.

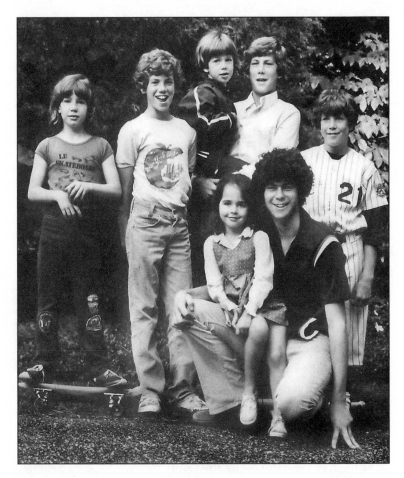

Standing: *Laurie Goldman, Scott Meltsner, Brian Meltsner holding Mike Goldman, and Danny Meltsner.* Front: *David Meltsner holding Sasha Kurtz, 1978.*

For years, Brenda's boys have attended Sea Gull, the brother camp of Seafarer. Which is, I'm sure, why Laurie wants to go. Just as I follow Brenda's lead, Laurie follows her cousins'. She plays the sports they play, wears a baseball cap every day like they do, terry wristband, no dresses. Of course, our two families are together constantly, at my house or Brenda's—birthdays, Rosh Hashanah lunch, Yom Kippur break-the-fast, Thanksgiving, the first night of Hanukkah, Passover, Mother's Day, Father's Day, even the Fourth of July. Thanksgiving, after dinner, the cousins go bowling. Many Sunday evenings, we meet for pizza. We take family trips together to the mountains and beach. We've traveled to California and England. (Brenda called one day, breathless. She'd found cheap tickets to London. "We've got to book seats this minute." We took the kids. Donald and Sasha joined us.) *Cousins* isn't a strong enough word for the connection between Brenda's children and mine.

She tells me to send in the reservation form for the camp bus (leaving from Charlotte) as soon as I receive it, that seats fill up quickly because everyone knows it's a great way for campers to meet *before* camp. Brenda's two youngest, Scott (twelve) and Danny (eleven), will be going this year (1979). She thinks the camp bus would be a good thing for Laurie, too.

The bus form arrives. I fill it out right on the mail table in the front hall and drive it to the post office. Brenda sends hers in a couple of days later.

Weeks pass. Brenda stops by my house to tell me that Scott and Danny did not get on the camp bus. Their applications arrived too late; every seat was taken. Laurie did get a seat.

"I have an idea," she says.

We're standing in my kitchen. Danny has joined Laurie and Mike in the backyard. Through the window over the sink, I can see Danny climbing along the top rail of the swing set. Laurie and Mike are right behind him. Now Danny is hanging by his knees, T-shirt sliding up, belly out, the knees of his jeans rubbed green from the wet grass. Laurie and Mike are hanging by their knees, too. The light through the trees runs over all of them carelessly.

"Why don't you cancel Laurie's reservation on the bus, and let's fly all three of them to camp?" Brenda says. "It's a short flight. They'll have to change planes in Raleigh, but then it's a straight shot to New Bern, and somebody from camp can pick them up and drive them to Arapahoe, or the kids could take a bus from New Bern to Arapahoe. Scott is old enough to be in charge of the two younger ones."

I turn toward her, concentrate on her face. Her skin is clear, flawless. "I don't know. . . . I'm not sure about that," I say. "What kind of bus?"

"Well, a Greyhound or Trailways."

I'm trying to imagine Scott looking out for Danny and Laurie. Scott and Danny can't spend ten minutes together without fighting. Not just fighting. I mean stitches, broken bones, heavy objects hurled across the room. I try to visualize the three of them changing planes in Raleigh, finding the gate, getting from the New Bern airport to the New Bern bus station, keeping up with their things, keeping up with *each other*.

I massage my temples with my fingers. Why did I ever agree to camp for Laurie in the first place?

"I just don't think Laurie's old enough to do all that," I finally say.

"You are so overprotective, Judy." She's suddenly stiff, head to toe. Clearly irked. "If you keep hovering, Laurie will never learn to be independent."

This is not the first time she's said something like this. She may be right, but I don't want to hear it from her.

"Well, our kids have never flown alone. Without us. Or done anything like this. And Laurie does have a seat on the camp bus . . . and anyway . . . just because I'm not sure . . ."

I'm opening the dishwasher and taking out glasses without checking to see if the machine has even run. Now the coffee mugs.

"You are impossible, Judy." A big sigh. "You are truly impossible."

I line up the glasses on the counter—juice glasses together, water glasses, mugs. The mugs have coffee drips down the sides. A couple of glasses have lipstick on the rims. I see that the knives and forks in the rack below are caked with food. Brenda is opening the back door, walking out, closing the door behind her hard—not exactly slamming it, just making sure *I* know it's shut. I hear her calling Danny to the car.

What I wish I could've said: *You have the right to ask, and I have the right to say no.* Which should be engraved on a plaque and presented to every older sister in America.

13

Later the same day, Brenda calls with another idea. Her voice is friendly again. Let's hire this young man, Frank (whom we both know superficially), to drive the three kids to camp.

She obviously has a higher opinion of Frank than I do. He has always seemed pretty unreliable to me. Not married, probably in his forties, he's active in local politics, ran for office several times, was never elected. When he's quoted in the paper, his remarks are off balance, often inflammatory.

"I don't know," I say, feeling a little off-balance myself. "He doesn't seem like the type of person we want to be in charge of our children. How well do you know him?"

"I know him well enough. My gosh, he ran for public office! You are *way* too tied in to your kids." She sounds thoroughly exasperated, as though she's told me this a thousand times and I haven't paid a bit of attention. "Let them grow up, Judy."

"Well . . ." Before I can get my sentence going, she's hung up.

I don't want to just sit here and take it. I feel a revving up in my chest. My hand reaches for the phone, and I imagine dialing her number, letting loose a chain of rough-edged words, then hanging up on *her*. But I stop myself before my finger touches the first button. Anger is not something I'm accustomed to feeling, and I'm certainly not good at showing it. Brenda's the one with the temper. "She comes by it naturally," Mother would say, in that way parents get impatient with offspring who exhibit the same hard-to-live-with traits of their husbands or wives.

My phone goes back in its cradle.

Anyway, this is not the time for me to confront Brenda. In addition to the worry she and I share over our parents, she has even bigger worries at home: three teenage boys, and the oldest, David, is rebelling in major ways. He was a precocious little boy—walked at nine months—and still has a dimply smile that wins your heart. But something is tugging at him, and he's cutting school, hanging out with the wrong crowd, following the Grateful Dead, saying and doing belligerently illogical things in that way that teenagers practically announce they're up to no good. Recently, he crashed his car into a tree in a secluded wooded area. When I drove Chuck out to pick up the car, we found pot and paraphernalia all over the front seat.

Why is Brenda so determined that I forgo the camp bus and send Laurie with her boys?

Maybe she feels stuck in having to find a ride for Scott and Danny, and she wants me to be more empathetic, join her. Maybe she's thinking, *Laurie got on the bus, but what about my kids? Doesn't Judy care how my kids get to camp?*

Which raises the question: Why *aren't* I being more empathetic? Why don't I join her in figuring out a way for all our kids to travel to camp together?

Truth is, I'm being just as determined as she is. She did tell me the camp bus is a good way for campers to meet, and I'm not only nervous about Laurie's adjustment to camp and eager to do whatever I can to help that along, I'm also used to taking my sister's advice. But are those the only motives at work here?

Am I just being stubborn?

Am I being overprotective? How dangerous would it be for three kids to fly together? And what if Frank is perfectly safe?

Maybe my dismissal of her fly-them-to-camp plan and her let-Frank-drive-them plan feels to her like a judgment. As though I'm saying she's not protective *enough* of her children. If she feels I'm criticizing her parenting, then naturally she has to come back with criticism of mine.

At the root of it all, of course, the subtext, the scribbling in the margins: Me, experimenting with something totally new in our relationship, raising a palm in protest. Seeing what it's like to make my own way.

Such unfamiliar territory for us. Little sister Judy not following big sister Brenda.

Of course, the situation—her life hard, mine not so hard—is very familiar. When Henry and I were newlyweds, Brenda and Chuck already had four boys, ranging from six down to newborn. Here's what evenings were like at their house: Brenda would be walking one baby, jiggling him, on her way to another baby, whose crying had reached unignorable levels. Chuck would pass her in the upstairs hall, on his way to one of the older boys.

How did Brenda save her sanity? She'd admired a small painting of flowers at a friend's house, but when she went to buy one for herself, she found it too expensive. *I'll just do my own,* she decided.

She bought canvases and acrylics and, in the midst of playpens and bibs stained orange from Gerber carrots, she taught herself to paint. It wasn't long before she had a number of canvases that were really lovely. She then bought remnants from framing shops, and she and Chuck framed the paintings themselves. On one of their buying trips to New York for the stores (he's in business with our father in Rock Hill, commutes from Charlotte), Chuck talked her into taking a suitcase of paintings to Henri Bendel. The buyer wanted every one. Their next trip to New York: Lord & Taylor, Bloomingdale's, Bonwit Teller. Soon she was selling to stores and galleries across the country.

Her boys are older now, and she's no longer painting

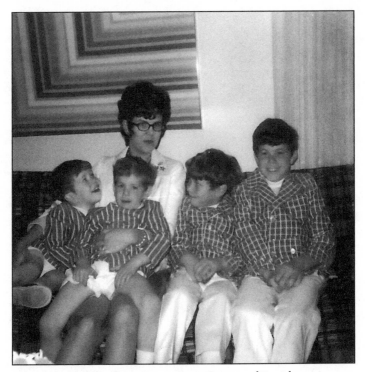

Brenda holding her boys, Danny, Scott, Brian, and David, 1970

miniatures. But life at home is again swallowing her up. She'll soon start a new business, airbrushing T-shirts. Then, after years of helping friends decorate their houses, she'll go into interior design.

For now, maybe she just wants to have something—one thing—settled.

Nervous about a daughter going away for five weeks, a daughter who can't spend the night out, I suppose I also want something—one thing—settled.

Camp turns into a subject my sister and I can't touch. Then no subject is safe. This seemingly insignificant dilemma—how to get our children from here to there—will lead to two years of Brenda barely speaking to me.

14

My father is weak and in pain, but intent on staying alive as long as Mother needs him. His pain intensifies. The doctors prescribe more radiation. Then a period of calm. Then more pain, more radiation, calm again. As though he keeps walking into traps, and stepping out.

Overnight, Mother's mind seems to have been jerked completely loose. She can't speak—she moans. She's lost control of her body—all she can do is writhe. My father, Brenda, and I take her to the hospital in Charlotte. The doctors say she probably suffered a stroke, maybe multiple strokes. Or they say it could be the Alzheimer's progressing. They tinker with her medications. At times, she lies there gazing vacantly, like a flounder washed onto the sand. Other times, she's more agitated than when we brought

her in, flinging herself from one side of the bed to the other, wail-
ing as if she doesn't know any other way to get help. Finally, the
doctors find the right balance. Though she's not exactly peaceful, she's no longer *so* agitated. The only awareness she shows is
when my father, Brenda, or I enters her hospital room and her
face lights up for that second.

She's about to be discharged from the hospital. My father has
said all along that when she's no longer aware of where she is, he'll
look into nursing homes. We all know that time has come. He
decides to look in Charlotte. I know what he's thinking: if Mother outlives him, he will have done everything possible to make it
easier for Brenda and me to care for her.

The three of us spend days checking out different places. I
don't say anything to my father about the rift between Brenda
and me. I can't tell if she has. What I do know is that he's totally
focused on finding a decent place for his beloved Peggy. Brenda is
acting like someone who dislikes me. She doesn't glance my way.
She hardly responds when I speak. When she speaks, it's to our
father. I alternate between watching every word—I don't want to
give her anything else to be mad at me about—and being envel-
oped by sadness at what we're getting ready to do with Mother.
Everything feels bunched up in my throat.

In the first nursing home, the smell of decay is so bad I gag.
The only way I can make it to the exit and fresh air is to unwrap
a stick of Juicy Fruit gum and hold it under my nose. In spite of
Brenda's upset with me, in spite of the dark circumstances (maybe *because* of the dark circumstances), we both laugh at what I'm
doing.

Of course, we've always been able to make each other laugh.
Years ago during a trip to New York, our parents took us to a
nightclub for an ice-skating show. At intermission, Brenda and

I left for the bathroom, found stalls side by side. I'd never seen anything so lavish. The stalls had wooden doors from floor to ceiling, and real doorknobs. Inside, it was like a tiny room. With wallpaper! I was so busy admiring my surroundings that I forgot to lift the lid. "Oh, no," Brenda heard me groan. She was immediately pulling at my door. I reached to unlock it. There I sat, my bare bottom in a pool of pee. She was practically falling on the floor. Both of us were helpless with laughter.

The next nursing home: Same smell as the first nursing home. Patients buzzing for help. Brenda and I lock eyes. We're both thinking, *Where are the nurses and aides? How are we going to do this?* We're not laughing anymore. But at least her anger has not returned. I don't know why it went away. I'm not asking any questions. I'm just relieved we're back to being two sisters, in sync, trying to do the right thing for our mother.

Next place: Sharon Towers. Quiet, clean, furnished like a historic home, with mahogany chests and vases of fresh flowers in the hallways, lamps casting a soft red glow. Brenda and I smile at each other. This is where we want Mother to be.

But they don't have a bed and can't say when one will become available.

We keep looking, find a place with an equally good reputation—and a vacancy. Wesley feels more like a hospital than Sharon Towers, but it's spotless and the nurses seem competent.

The next morning, we transfer Mother from the hospital to Wesley. Late afternoon, Sharon Towers calls to inform me they have a bed. I dial Brenda. "Whoever just died," I say, "died a day too late for us." She laughs, I laugh, a little more talk, but then the chill is back. Conversation over. I guess we've done what we had to do for Mother and can resume our fight.

When we happen to visit her on the same day, Brenda directs all her conversation to the nurses. Any phone calls between us are about driving our father to radiation, and they're strictly business.

"Can you do it today, Brenda?"

"Yes."

Or "It's your turn, Judy."

"I know."

One day, I'm wheeling Mother around her floor, which always, whether it's mealtime or not, smells like custard. Wheelchair patients line the hall, most of them around the nurses' station, where trays high on the counter hold tiny paper cups of pills. The patients, mostly women, don't change their expressions when we pass by. Suddenly, Mother starts waving to each person, blowing kisses, as though it's her job to cheer the place up. I'm thrilled with this renewed awareness, a gesture so typical of the old her.

But then, just as quickly as it appeared, it disappears. No more awareness. No moaning either, which is a relief. But no sounds at all. No memory left of the "old her" anywhere in her body.

Something else, totally crazy and not easy to admit: I want to wash my hands every time I touch her. Get the Alzheimer's off me. If she can succumb to a disease like this—someone who's so beautiful, so important—anyone can. The barrier between me and *it* has developed huge cracks and can cave in any moment. However, if I lather down to the base of each finger, if I lather up to my wrists, I can separate myself—at least where this disease is concerned—from Mother.

15

My father worries about burdening Brenda and me, but staying in Charlotte with either of us means he can go to the nursing home early in the morning and sit beside Mother's bed till dark. He's not physically strong enough to drive the twenty-six miles between Rock Hill and Charlotte.

He moves in with Brenda. After several weeks, she tells me she thinks it's time for him to move to my house; she needs a break. That's okay with me. Our conversation is brief. It accomplishes what it needs to accomplish.

After breakfast one morning, my father and I are in my kitchen. I'm peeling potatoes for split pea and barley soup, Mattie's recipe. Whenever I make it, I picture her in the kitchen on Eden Terrace, potato peels flying off her quick fingers.

My pot, on the counter next to the sink, is filled with water. I've already plopped in the carrots, onions, celery, soup bone, split peas, and barley. My father is at the kitchen table reading the morning paper. He turns toward me, holding his neck at a funny angle. I can tell it hurts. "I want to buy you a present, Judy. Something you would never buy for yourself. It's the only way I'll feel okay about staying here."

"You don't need to do that," I say. "I love having you."

"No, no. How about furniture for your living room? A sofa. Or a pair of chairs. Think big."

"Well, it's interesting you're asking me this. Last night, I dreamed I was buying a desk. But instead of taking the time to find the right desk, I settled for the first one I found. And the cheapest. An ugly, modern one with a Formica top."

"So what would your ideal desk be?" He's turning into Mother. He listens now, asks questions. He's becoming sensitive. Chatty. If the other person thinks a subject is important, then it's important. As though Mother moved out and he moved in. Everyone in the family has noticed the change. Every February for years, my parents and Mother's younger sister, Aunt Katie, and her husband spent three weeks on the west coast of Florida. My father and Uncle Irwin have always considered themselves best friends. The two of them would sit in the shade and read for hours, not uttering a word. Later, they would say they'd had the time of their lives. Now, Uncle Irwin says with a smile, he can't get off the phone when Bennie calls.

"My ideal desk would be too expensive," I answer. "An old roll-top, the kind with all those cubbyholes and drawers and pull-out things. But any nice wooden desk would be great—"

"A roll-top is what I want you to have," he says. He reaches into his shirt pocket, then waves a check. I can see from across the room it's already made out. For a thousand dollars! I nearly fall in the soup.

Weeks later, Henry and I are in New York for a Goldman

cousin's wedding. We spend every free minute shopping for a desk in the Village, in and out of shadowy antique stores, until we find the desk of my dreams on Perry Street—a golden oak S-curve roll-top, cubbies in all shapes and sizes, large dovetailed drawers, two tiny hidden pencil drawers, pull-out writing boards, solid raised side panels, five feet wide, four feet tall, ornate brass plaque right in the front (*Indianapolis Cabinet Company*), late nineteenth century, perfect condition, the wood smooth as bone.

It's the last present my father will give me.

16

My father has been at my house for several weeks.

One night after he's in bed, I call Brenda. "Do you think Daddy could come back to your house?" I ask. "I'm feeling like I need a break."

"You do know, Judy"—that tone of voice—"I'm carrying more than my share of the burden."

"Well," I say, thinking a recital of the facts will straighten out whatever this new misunderstanding is about, "he started out at your house, and then you told me you needed a break, so he moved to my house. I'm only asking for the same thing you asked for."

"You have never been able to handle difficult things. He hasn't even been at your house that long. I knew you'd need him to leave as soon as he got there."

"That's not true, Brenda. He's been at my house the same

amount of time he was at your house. I'm just saying let's take turns and keep track of the time."

"This isn't about taking turns. You're not doing your part. But that's perfectly all right. He can come back here. And you know what? He doesn't have to come back to your house at all. Ever."

"Brenda, that's not what I want. If you'd just—"

But the angrier person gets to decide when the conversation is over.

I'm still holding the phone. I turn toward the window over the kitchen sink and look at the stars, how they've locked themselves into place.

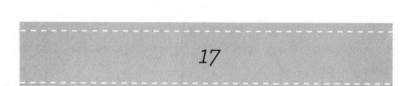

17

The next day, Aunt Emma, Mother's older sister, calls. We chat a little, but I suspect we haven't gotten to the real purpose of the call.

"I was talking to Brenda," she says. "She told me you're having a hard time with your father at your house. She says it's too much for you."

In our family, we don't just have parent/daughter teams. We also have aunt/niece teams. Aunt Emma's daughter is near Brenda's age, so Aunt Emma and Brenda are close. Aunt Katie's daughter and I are almost the same age, so Aunt Katie (who died several years ago) and I were close. Of course, there's always been great affection between Aunt Emma and me, between Aunt Katie and Brenda; it's just that, for all those childhood visits in Columbia with our cousins, I stayed at Aunt Katie's house, Brenda at Aunt Emma's.

I hear myself answering jaggedly, "Oh, no . . . That's not it. . . . I was happy to have him. . . . It was fine. . . . Brenda just . . . And Daddy . . . Well, I told Brenda . . ."

I feel tears in my eyes. Does my failure to manage this conversation confirm that I failed to manage my father's stay?

"Darling Judy, you're just like your mother," Aunt Emma says. "So very sweet. You're both as sweet as you can be. Just not strong. Your mother had a hard time handling difficult things, too."

I used to like being told that I was the sweet one and Brenda the strong one. But I don't want to hear that now. Yes, I'm having trouble coping. But so is Brenda. She's not being any braver than I am. And Aunt Emma is not criticizing just me, she's criticizing Mother. Where is the truth about those three sisters? I never heard one unfavorable remark from Mother about Aunt Emma or Aunt Katie—the story has always been how attached they were. What *were* the dynamics among them? Did Mother want Brenda and me to accomplish what she and her sisters could not? Is what's going on between Brenda and me somehow *inevitable*?

Brenda *was* the strong one. She was so strong I made her my guide, measured myself against her. And I *was* the sweet one. She could count on me to admire her, follow her lead, do whatever I had to do to keep things smooth between us. Our temperamental differences gave our relationship its power. Our defining roles were our adhesive.

My father ends up returning to Brenda's house. How this happens is lost to me soon after he moves. Standing up to my sister feels so dangerous that all the details quickly vanish.

Brenda and I were planning a trip together this summer to visit Donald and Mara at their weekend house in the Hamptons. I assume we're still going. Maybe a vacation will heal us.

But Brenda calls to say she doesn't think it's a good idea for us to go together, she'll go without me because her life is hard right now and she really needs to get away, I should just cancel my ticket.

I feel myself shrinking back into my old self. I call the airline.

18

Days before camp, Chuck tells me he and Brenda are going to drive Scott and Danny to Camp Sea Gull.

Henry and I, on a rain-slicked morning, take Laurie to a high-school parking lot on the other side of town, where she'll board the camp bus.

The driver loads Laurie's trunk, which she has artfully decorated with stickers, into the luggage bin. Bravely, she kisses us good-bye, climbs the steep steps, does not turn around for a wave or even a last look.

She finds a window seat near the front. The seat beside her is empty. As the bus snorts and coughs its way out into traffic, Henry and I wave enthusiastically, both of us with two hands, as though we're trying to teach an infant how to do bye-bye. I glance from the front of the bus to the back. She's the only one not sitting—and chattering and laughing—with a friend. She presses her forehead to the window. I can see tears streaming down her cheeks.

She starts to wave. Soon her lifted hand is blurry with waving.

Exactly what I feared: that she would take this adventure-some step—a step she might not be ready for—and it would overwhelm her. Why didn't I just let her fly with her cousins? At least she wouldn't be alone. And Brenda and I would still be okay. I want to pluck Laurie from her seat and deposit her back in my car. *Bad idea, honey. Let's go home.*

But I don't move. I stand here, in this drizzle of a morning, under a long sky, waving.

Laurie is homesick the first few days, adjusts, is homesick again when we leave after visitors' day, adjusts, loves camp, returns every summer for years, becomes a junior counselor, then counselor. Her feelings about camp could not be more different from what I'd feared.

What caused this deep fracture between Brenda and me?
Her turmoil at home?
My lack of empathy?
My asking if our father could move back?
Her temper?
My nervousness over Laurie and camp?
I go back and forth between blaming her and blaming myself. What I don't yet know is that it's really neither her fault nor mine. There are many tentacles.

Our parents are dying, and we each want the other to take away the pain.
Make me feel better, Brenda.
Make me feel better, Judy.
When neither of us can, we do the only thing we *can* do: turn on each other.

Also, something else: our parents would never have permitted this falling-out. Not that they would have interfered; they weren't the type to knowingly direct our lives. But Mother believed in the sister bond, and our father loved her beyond all reason and therefore supported her. Even though they were far from heavy-handed, we knew their feelings. I suddenly rebel, go against our parents by *not* going along with my sister—and she dishes out consequences for my actions. Our parents should be steering us back onto the path. But they're not here.

Without our parents—without parents the way they're supposed to be (healthy, participating)—my sister and I are totally lost. We loved the parallel tracks we were on, our prescribed roles in the family, our Mother/Judy, Daddy/Brenda teams. With nobody telling us who we are, everything is up for grabs.

I stand up to Brenda, show her I can tolerate distance between us—*I'm suddenly strong! I'm no longer sweet! I don't even care how you get your kids to camp!*—and neither of us knows what to do with the new Judy. Brenda is furious at my reversal. Her anger scares me to death.

Dealing with her rebelling son at the same time she's losing both parents, Brenda must feel deeply vulnerable. Brenda vulnerable? That would scare *both* of us.

I can't believe what has happened to my sister and me. I'm steeped in sadness. At times, I allow myself to be angry. Deep down, I miss her.

19

Donald, on the phone one night, makes a suggestion I never would have expected.

"How 'bout if I try to mediate between you and Brenda? I think I might be able to help you two work this out." He's coming to Charlotte soon.

All along, he has stayed neutral. Painstakingly neutral. The few times he allowed himself to enter into a conversation with me about Brenda, I tried to make him take my side, but he would not. I have a feeling the same thing happens when she talks to him about me. We both would love for him to be the final judge, love to be the one declared right.

I also would love for him to help us end this.

Since he's staying with Brenda and Chuck, we make a plan to meet at their house after dinner. Our father will be back home in Rock Hill that evening.

I ask Henry to accompany me. He's not sure it's a good idea.

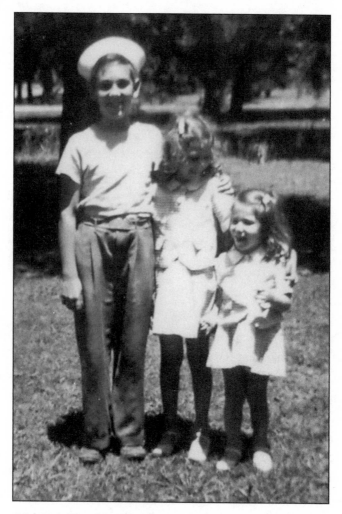

With Donald and Brenda, 1944

"But Chuck will be there," I say, "and I don't want to have to go up against Brenda *and* Chuck. I'll feel safer if you're there."

Henry is sturdy and confident, the kind of person you can grab onto. "Well," he says, "of course I'll go . . . if it'll make you feel better." He's also sensitive. Our friends say that of all the husbands in our group, he's the "most evolved," the one whose feminine sensibility is the most highly developed. It's a standing joke among us but also true. In the light pouring down on him from the lamp beside his chair, his eyes couldn't be browner. "I don't think I should join in the conversation, though, since this is between you and Brenda."

"I agree. But just having you there . . ."

Sure enough, when we walk in, Chuck is next to Brenda on the sectional in the den. Donald is off to the side in a chair that used to belong to Chuck's mother. Henry and I take the short end of the sofa.

Brenda and I sit very upright. Her knees point out. My knees point toward her.

Donald says something introductory that he probably thought out ahead of time—something about his hopes that this thing can be resolved, that he feels he's the one, because of his unique position in the family, who might be able to make it happen. I hear the dishwasher thrumming in the kitchen. Chuck looks away for a moment. Henry does, too. Brenda and I don't move. All four of our knees stay pointed.

Brenda starts talking. Her voice is taut with anger, which makes me feel hopeless. And nervous. And, not able to think straight. How can I stay clear? My hands tighten in my lap. Mostly, I stare dumbly at the carpet. My breath is coming in such short huffs that when I speak, I say only a few words at a time.

Donald is careful not to interrupt either of us, although I sense him trying, unsuccessfully, to guide. He asks for more precise explanations of what really happened at certain points. He obviously had no idea what he was volunteering for, how deep the divide. Chuck and Henry remain silent.

Finally, Donald's face lights up with irritation and he says, "Brenda, you are being so defensive, it makes me rise up out of my chair. And Judy, you're being so silent, I don't see how this is ever going to be resolved."

The rest is gone from my memory—how we respond to him, *if* we respond, who says what next. One thing is clear: Donald can't take the place of our parents. We need one of them sitting in that carved mahogany chair across from us.

Another thing I know for sure is that the last words are Brenda's, and they're spoken to me: "We're just so very different, Judy."

As though she's delivering the closing argument. And there's nothing more for any of us to say.

Chuck lets Henry and me out the door. We walk through the garage, around their cars, to our car parked in the driveway beside Brenda's vegetable garden. My face feels red.

Henry and I talk a little on the way home. What's playing over and over in my mind is her last statement. Those words suddenly carry more weight than ever before. I believe she's saying, *You should be more like me.* Which I then take a step farther: *But you're not like me. You're less than me.* Which I then take to: *If you were more like me, we might have a chance.* Ending with: *We're so different, there is no way we can ever have a relationship.*

Just before sleep, I push all that away and try to think how I could have made the evening go better.

Middle of the night, I wake and it dawns on me, the way I always think of precisely the right comeback, only much too late. Well, it's not exactly a comeback I think of. It's a way I might have kept the conversation going.

Why didn't I simply accept what she said? We *are* very different.

What if I had entered into a conversation about how different we are? Such an ordinary thing, to acknowledge the other's otherness. That's Brenda being Brenda, that's Judy being Judy, that's Judy trying not to be Judy, Brenda trying not to be Brenda, the two of us following the pattern, breaking the pattern, why couldn't I just deal with the complexity, no wonder we get confused, we need to lean back and look around, be grateful we can sit together, try to understand the follies of each person reacting to the way the world works, our cranky differences, what is it that's so difficult, come on now.

20

Weeks after our failed summit, I call Brenda to propose that the two of us see a therapist. Someone who is *not* our brother.

We've each been in therapy for months. I started going because I couldn't face losing my parents. Now I spend more time talking about losing my sister. I'm seeing Paula. She's seeing Rick. When Brenda says okay, I ask which therapist she'd rather us see. How about Rick? she says. I stop seeing Paula and start seeing Rick so I can establish a rapport with him before we see him together.

When the day arrives, we drive in separate cars. No mention of either of us swinging by for the other. In the waiting room, we read magazines. Rick appears in the doorway to call us back. We follow solemnly, as though we're entering a room where we'll select our parents' caskets.

He starts with me, raising questions. I answer carefully, tentatively. He responds kindly to what I say, lets me know he understands. He makes suggestions for how I might react differently. So far, so good.

Now it's Brenda's turn. He asks her questions. She answers angrily. He listens, responds kindly, lets her know he understands. She says more—angry, angry. He makes suggestions for how she might react differently. She stands, slings her purse over her shoulder, looks at him with that look I've seen before, and says, "I don't have to sit here and take this."

And she stalks out.

I stare at the door in disbelief. With an awful suddenness (and not a small amount of self-righteousness), I picture my underwear strewn across the front yard on Eden Terrace—the cotton underpants a six- or seven-year-old would wear, my undershirts and socks. Brenda, enraged at something I'd said or done, had raised the second-floor window of our room, unlatched the screen, pulled out my dresser drawer and dumped the entire contents onto the grass, like litter, for all the neighborhood to see.

I remember the times she ran away from home. The suitcases she packed and lugged down the stairs. The Last Will & Testaments she drew up. (Once, angry with Mother, Brenda willed all her stuffed animals to me. I hated to see her go but was happy with what I got.)

I turn to Rick, whose eyes are closed so tight you'd think he might break them. I'm glad to have a witness to Brenda's temper. But then he looks straight at me and says something I don't want to hear: "Judy, I think you're going to have to bury the relationship."

I go silent. Everything that went on prior to this second is suddenly outside of words. I cannot remember a thing.

He seems to sense this and offers, "To Brenda, that must have felt like a dentist probing."

Finally, I speak. "Do you think she didn't want to be here in the first place?"

"It's possible," he says. "Sometimes, a decision is made, and you're just waiting for the data to support it. Decisions can be made unawares, and then you accumulate injustices."

Keep going, I'm thinking.

He says that the expression on my face while she was talking was one of shock, as though I knew things were not right between us but had no idea how not-right they really were.

"I could see your mouth was open, Judy, but no words were coming."

I glance around the room, remember that he once told me Brenda had given him suggestions for rearranging the furniture. I wonder if this is the original grouping or what she'd thought would work better. He laughed warm-heartedly when he told me she was his first client to make interior design suggestions.

Now he's saying it's obvious I believed this was fixable. The word he uses to describe me is *naïve*. Some things, he tells me, are not fixable. Just because you have a problem doesn't mean you have a solution.

The first time I met with Rick, I told him I had a charmed childhood. He refers to this and says that early childhood experiences, if benign, don't require the development of certain skills, which means the skills are late in coming. Acceptance is also late in coming. "You're not accustomed to failure, Judy, not practiced at it." He says my request for a repair of the relationship was reasonable. But given the circumstances, not realistic.

"Okay," I say. And after a few seconds: "Okay." And then: "I get it." It's those skills Aunt Emma sees in Brenda and the absence of those skills she sees in me. It's the satin pillow I'm still resting on.

The first time I called Rick to make an appointment, he re-

marked how identical Brenda and I sounded on the phone. Now
he's telling me how different we are. The wounds in our relationship are what he's focusing on, how he sees the wounds more vo-
cally in Brenda, she's quicker.

He calls her the externalizer; me, the internalizer.

"What does that mean?" I ask.

"Are you spurting blood?" he says. "Or are you hemorrhaging
internally?"

I swallow. Those images—so opposite, so the same. Here it is:
Brenda is hurting as much as I am. Maybe more.

"Your sister is overly sensitive to external cues. She as-
cribes too much to them. You're overly sensitive to your internal states, Judy. One is not better or worse than the other.
They're just different."

Years from now, I'll look up these terms: People with internal
locus of control (internalizers, like me) feel they have the power
to do something about a situation. They blame themselves for
personal actions that go wrong and take credit for the ones that
go well. People with external locus of control (externalizers, like
Brenda) believe events are caused by factors beyond their control. They tend to be fatalistic, crediting circumstances or fate for
the good in their lives, blaming outside forces for the bad. When
problems occur, externalizers (because they feel a lack of control)
will not try to repair relationships.

"So what would you say my part is in all this?" I ask.

"Your tenacity," he answers. "How desperately you want reso-
lution. You're like a Weeble. You know those roly-poly toys?
You wobble, but you don't fall down. You just keep trying.
It wouldn't surprise me if your doggedness comes across to
Brenda as aggressive."

"What is Brenda's part?" I ask.

"A distorted lens through which she sees herself as ever the aggrieved party. No matter what happens, some people find the cloud behind every silver lining. None of us can ever know another person's intentions, so we respond to their behavior by *ascribing* intentions to them. If we feel coerced or threatened, we ascribe malice to the other person. Brenda is looking out for the traps. Anything you say can be held against you."

"That's exactly what it feels like." I don't mind hearing him point out her flaws.

I glance at the clock. Out of time. One final question: "How do you see the two of us?"

Without hesitating, he answers, "Cain and Abel." I make a mental note to read the Bible story again.

His wrap-up: Give up. My attempts at repair will only be interpreted negatively. I need to stop asking for something I won't get. The opportunity costs are too high. I need to spend my energy more profitably. Mourn certain hopes.

For my next session, which, obviously, will be alone, he instructs me to bring in something that represents Brenda, something with deep meaning, and we will bury it in the ground, behind his office.

This is one of the hardest tasks I've ever been given. A term paper, even a doctoral dissertation, would be a piece of cake compared to this. After rifling through my jewelry box, my dresser, my closet, I select a pinkish scarf hand-knit in the North Carolina mountains. Brenda gave it to me years ago for my birthday. She couldn't decide whether to give me the scarf or a copy of *Maida Heatter's Book of Great Desserts*, so she showed me both and told me to pick. When I had a hard time deciding, she gave me the scarf and the book.

The day of my therapy appointment, I fold the scarf back onto my closet shelf.

Now I'm panicked. The good student in me wants to complete the assignment, make a good grade. But what to take?

I grab from the wall going up the stairs a photograph of the two of us we had taken for Mother on Mother's Day. I was in junior

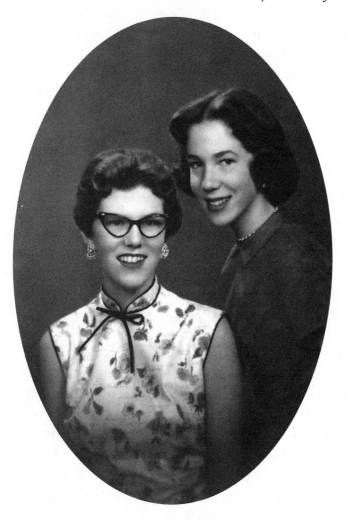

Photo of Brenda and me taken for Mother's Day, 1955

high, Brenda in high school. I still remember the dresses we wore. Mine was aqua and low waisted. Hers was a creamy cotton with pastel flowers, trimmed in thin black ribbon.

No, I can't do it. I can't give up this picture. I don't want to bury the relationship. What I want is my sister. I hang the photograph of Brenda and me back on the wall, pat it into place.

I end up bringing an unimportant letter she wrote to me in college, the only one I wouldn't mind sacrificing. It's short, doesn't say anything noteworthy. When I hand it to Rick, he reads it, smiles, gives it back to me. "I see you're not ready to let go," he says. "I thought we might do something ritualistic that would not only reflect the feelings but create the feelings. It's okay. We've got a little more work to do."

Like our father, Brenda knows how to bury relationships. Years ago, he did the same with *his* sister. His *twin* sister.

Imagine—twins, married, with families of their own, living in small-town Rock Hill, blocks apart, one having nothing to do with the other. The disagreement was over money. I once overheard Mother urging Daddy to mend the rift, Daddy wanting nothing more to do with his twin sister. "I've lost respect for her," I heard him say matter-of-factly.

Most people in Rock Hill didn't even know we were related. My main memory of Aunt Sarah is actually of her husband, Uncle Morris, and it's a very slim memory. Every December, he played the xylophone on the Shriners' float in the Christmas parade. One year, the float stopped right in front of where I was standing. In a split second, he signaled to me; I jumped on. He handed me his mallets, and I started playing: *Over hill, over dale, we will hit the dusty trail, as those caissons go rolling along.* It was all so exotic—having an uncle who wore a fez, having an uncle who was a musician, having an uncle I barely knew—the two of us cruising down Main Street like entertainers on an ocean liner.

It's a truth I know but don't want to know: there's a crack down the middle of my relationship with Brenda large enough for generations of sisters to fall through.

21

I have a million conversations with Brenda. In the shower. Driving in the car, running errands, standing in line at the grocery store. At 3 A.M. They undo my hesitant attempt at independence, my defying her. They undo her stern reaction.

Yes, I say, *all sisters are different. As individual as thumbprints. But . . .*

That's when she interrupts me: *But . . . we're sisters.*

Then we talk everything over, see each other's side, make up.

In real life, though, we hardly speak.

I could easily take to my bed. Instead, I take to my typewriter. I write poem after maudlin poem about losing my sister, losing my parents, losing my brother (who's again staying as far away as possible). In one sweep, I've lost the family I grew up in. Writing is my way of admitting I cannot rearrange life.

Writing *poetry* is my way of making sure that nothing I put down on paper will ever be read by my sister. If a poem does get published in a literary journal, the only people who'll read it are other poets. If the poem is especially revealing about the two of us, I won't even submit it to poetry journals. I'll hide it in the bottom drawer of my desk. It will be as if the words dissolved on my tongue.

22

Last Night

It was late enough to see a luna moth.
From where I stood I could watch
it wave, such quick flicks of wing
you'd think the moon was pulling strings,
knuckling that small body
as if it were the immaculate hand of a magician
turning a silk scarf into gardenias,
into something that flies,
into a sister determined to move so far away
I can only stand in the unmowed grass
watching the sky, the one thing left
we have in common.

23

It's the day before Thanksgiving, late 1940s or early 1950s. The year doesn't matter because the scene replays every November: Mother is balancing on a wooden stepladder with a bucket of sudsy ammonia water, taking apart the chandelier over the dining-room table, one crystal at a time, washing each as if it were a diamond earring. My father is at work, Donald and Brenda somewhere in the neighborhood. I hear Mattie in the kitchen, chopping celery and onions for her cornbread dressing, singing along with the radio, her gospel hymns Jesusing through the house. I'm sitting at the head of the table in my father's uphol-stered wing chair, legs dangling. I picture the jewel in Mother's hand hanging from my ear.

Now it's November 1979, the night before Thanksgiving (not long after Brenda's and my joint-therapy session). I dream the following:

I'm lost in the cold, bare-walled basement of a hospital or nursing home. I'm just about to find my way out when rusty water spurts from a faucet in the commercial-style sink. Thinking fast, I put out my cigarette and pull a small towel from my purse to sop up the foul-smelling water before it can overflow from the countertop onto the floor. Good. All taken care of. Again, I turn to leave. More water spurts out. Then it surges, gushing over the counter, onto the floor, into the corridor. *Thank goodness I'm wearing sneakers, not dress shoes,* I say to myself. But within minutes, the rancid water is up to my knees. I slosh out into the hall and encounter a man—obviously a patient, old and frail. He asks me to get him a chair. *How can I possibly do what he wants when I already have so much to deal with? If I can just find Henry, he'll help me clean up this mess.*

The dream is not hard to analyze. Brenda and I are barely speaking; everything is stalled between us. Our father is growing weaker. Mother, in the final stages of Alzheimer's, in the nursing home, doesn't know anyone, can't engage at all—her eyes have gone flat. Over and over, eye doctor Henry moves his hand in front of her face, looking for a sign that she's aware of the shadow. Over and over, he turns to me, his eyebrows squeezed together in the middle of his forehead, his mouth twisted sadly to the side.

I fantasize combining my mother's body with my father's brain. One healthy body + one healthy brain = one complete parent.

One complete parent = Brenda + Judy.

Here's what Mother was like before: She didn't just walk. She sprang forward, light as air, each step a rise on the balls of her feet, as though she were moving toward something that would prove too thrilling to even think of missing.

Everyone loved her. If you admired something of hers, she gave it to you. At Christmas, she delivered poinsettias all over town, to friends, acquaintances, people who didn't fit either of those categories: Teachers whom Donald, Brenda, and I had, present and past. The woman who checked out our books at the public library. The elderly blind man who operated the steel, cagelike elevator in the People's Bank building, who every summer brought Mother shoeboxes of homegrown vegetables. One Christmas, I went with her to the Catawba Indian Reservation to deliver a poinsettia to a family she'd sat beside once at the soda fountain in the drugstore.

She was optimistic, and trusted the good in others. Her antidote to anti-Semitism: Jews should not be clannish. If non-Jewish people could just get to know us, one by one, they would see that we are regular, ordinary people. When Brenda and I were confirmed, Mother convinced the other Jewish parents to invite neighbors, friends, their children's schoolmates and teachers, even near-strangers to the ceremony. She wanted the entire town to see firsthand how important family is to us all, how parents just want their children to continue the traditions of their religion, how very much alike we all are.

After I married and was living in Charlotte, I never went to see her without finding her standing at the top of the driveway, waiting for my car to turn in. Before I left for home, she'd fill my arms with steaks cut extra thick and wrapped for the freezer, summer peaches, tomatoes, a chicken pie fresh-baked by Mattie. I'd zigzag my way down the long driveway, knowing that Mother would stand there waving until I'd driven past the fourteenth green, which was across the street and down the hill. Only then would she turn and go back in.

Here's what my father was like: A passionate businessman and golfer, he was nuts-and-bolts determined. He could be churlish; he did not suffer fools gladly. In fact, he prided himself on always speaking his mind. But he could be counted on to be fair. And stalwart.

Now here he is, so thin you can see the stringy veins beneath the skin on his face. He has trouble walking and sitting, is almost bald from the radiation on his face and skull, which we're hoping will keep his left cheek from hanging so limp.

Here is our father, saying he wants to have Thanksgiving at his house this year.

Understand, he never cooked a thing in his life. He was totally uninvolved in any holiday preparation, in any jobs having to do with the house. I never saw him carry a plate into the kitchen, never saw him rinse a glass. My father is offering to have Thanksgiving for the entire family—Brenda and Chuck and their four sons, Henry and me and our two kids, and Mattie. Donald (now separated from his wife) and daughter Sasha will fly down from New York. I understand my father's motivation: he knows Mother was happiest when the family was gathered in the house. Of course, she won't be here this year, but it's something he has to do.

Mattie does the cooking. But she and my father together do the shopping, set the table, even arrange the flowers. She later tells Brenda and me how he paid attention to every detail. "Can you believe cranberry sauce is forty-nine cents a can?" he said to her. "That's too expensive! Forget the A&P. We'll do better at Community Cash." And: "The sweet potatoes look good, don't you think, Mattie? The string beans are nice and fresh."

My father? Admiring produce?

Thanksgiving turns out to be another of those times when nerve endings are especially close to the surface, when it feels as though the earth itself has shifted. It's as though we've made a silent pact to pretend Daddy is healthy and Mother is here, to pretend Brenda and I are getting along. (Our kids are the biggest pretenders of all. They're desperate for their mothers to be "back to normal.") She and I move effortlessly through the kitchen helping Mattie, into the living room, onto the sofa beside each other to join the others in telling happy-to-be-here stories.

My father knows—Mattie, Brenda and her family, Donald and Sasha, my family and I know—this is the last time we'll all be together in this house.

Here's what the days leading up to Thanksgiving 1979 are like for me:

Laurie and Mike are ten and seven, my advertising copywriting business is as busy as ever, I try to visit Mother three or four times a week, Brenda and I, using few words, work out taking turns driving our father to radiation. Before Thanksgiving, a routine chest x-ray reveals a spot on my mother-in-law's lung, which turns out to be malignant. She recuperates from surgery at our house.

There is not enough of me to go around. How can I possibly find the time to direct a school play, which Laurie's fifth-grade teacher says will help her adjust to her new school? We just moved her from a public open school (where students sat in real wooden boats or on the floor, instead of in chairs at desks) to a very traditional and academic private school. She has never done homework or taken tests. Then there are Mike's soccer practices and games. The team dinner at our house. Basketball season starts soon. I need to buy and wrap gifts, bring down Hanukkah decorations from the attic, address cards.

Cold, rusty water is rising faster than I can sop it up.

But Thanksgiving Day, when our family gathers in my parents' dining room, when my father slides the wing chair in at the head of the table, when Chuck carves the turkey, Brenda serves the rice and I ladle the gravy, Mattie cuts the cornbread dressing,

Henry passes the string beans and digs into the sweet potatoes,
Donald pours the iced tea and tells a funny joke and the children
poke each other because it's slightly off-color—the sun through
the windows turns everything golden and the rise of warmth in
the room is all we know.

24

I'm writing more and more poems. They're being published in literary journals. I'm teaching in Poetry-in-the-Schools, leading poetry workshops in adult education at a nearby college and at writers' conferences.

I give a reading in a bookstore in downtown Asheville, North Carolina. Before I begin the first poem, I say to the audience, mostly women, some students in workshops I've taught, most my age, mid-thirties, a few older: "I have never smoked a cigarette in my life. When I was little, though, I made a study of the way my mother held a cigarette. I'd practice for hours in front of the mirror, one arm folded across my middle, the elbow of the other cupped in my palm. Every now and then, I'd pick an imaginary fleck of tobacco off my tongue. Now here's the peculiar part: if

you looked in on my dreams now, you would see me holding a cigarette. I don't mean in occasional dreams. I mean in *every* dream."

In Dreams I'm Always Smoking

In dreams I'm always smoking
and I, lover of clean lungs
and sweet breath, laugh at the folly
of caution. Isn't it charming
the way I rest my elbow on the table,
my fingers curled back holding the cigarette
as if that part of me, from my wrist
to my fingertips, were a delicate Japanese drawing,
the cigarette only the tight wing
of a blossom. I bring it close to my face,
narrow my eyes when thin sheets of smoke
begin to cut, purse my lips
as if I were whispering the words to a song,
and then pulling in, everything,
believing it cool as the night air
that washes my face when I stand at the kitchen sink,
the window open, no screen.
I feel the smoke roll over my tongue,
spoonfuls of whipped pudding, and of course
in this part of the dream I inhale
pale grey down my throat,
pump it to places so deep in myself
it feels like something thin and light and slow
spilling over me, and to think
it all started with fire.

Before I read the next poem, I ask for a show of hands: "How many of you write poetry? Okay, here's an exercise for you to try. Picture your family of origin. Put them in an enclosed space—around a kitchen table, for example, or in a car. It's the old elevator trick; nobody's going anywhere. Now write your poem and suggest—without naming—the emotional climate. What does the air feel like?"

Sunday Night, Driving Home

If I close one eye the light from the dial
looks like the tip of a cigarette.
And my mother *is* smoking,
the small fingers of her left hand moving
to her lips, then to the curve of the front seat
close to my father's shoulder.
Her hand is a pigeon
in the shadows that fly in from the road.
My sister and I lie across the back seat,
our shoes touching, each of us resting
on a pillow pressed to the glass.
I think my sister is sleeping.
She's missing the talk from the front seat,
Aunt Katie said this—Aunt Emma, that. My father
offers an opinion. Mother appears to nod
instead of saying the word yes.
I hear less and less of their low tones
until suddenly the sound of wheels spinning gravel
and I know without opening my eyes
we are home. I also know that our father
will first lift my sister and carry her in,

return for me, placing me lightly
in the narrow bed next to hers,
folding the sheet back over the quilt
and smoothing it flat with the palm of his hand.
Then he'll touch my face, listen to me breathe
and reach for the switch on the lamp
that separates our twin beds
like the tall brass branch of a family tree.

After my reading, during the Q&A, a woman in the front
row raises her hand and offers shyly, a soft cadence to her voice, "I
think I know why you smoke in your dreams."

"You do?" I say.

"It's your mother," she says.

My mother. Yes. The woman is right. I've never read these
two poems aloud back to back, so I have never made that connection. Of course it's my mother. Day by day, I'm losing her in
slow circles, so I take little test runs to see what it will be like to
exist without her, *outside* her. In sleep, though, I keep her well and
normal by inhabiting her body.

Let's both be you.

Let's smoke.

25

Donald has brought Chris, his sunny, bouncy new girlfriend, down to meet us. They're staying with Henry and me. It's December 29, 1979, one month since Thanksgiving, two weeks since we found out our father's cancer has spread to his brain. (Now we know why the left side of his face droops.) He's suddenly so weak he can't get out of bed without help, so weak he can't control his bladder and bowels. He's at Brenda's.

Yesterday Brenda called Henry to come over to help clean up our father after he had an accident in the bed. Chuck was working; it was Henry's afternoon off.

Our father is sleeping, and Donald and Chris, Brenda and Chuck, Mattie, Henry and I are in Brenda and Chuck's living room trying to decide what's next. (These days, Mattie is spending a lot of time in Charlotte with Brenda or me, also.) Brenda pushes her glasses up, rubs her eyes, small grinding motions. For a second, I imagine her twirling her hair, the way she used to when she was young. She says our father is really too sick to be at home. She doesn't know how she'll take care of him now, doesn't know how she'll keep him comfortable. More important, she believes he feels humiliated having accidents. He had another one last night, and Chuck took him into the shower.

Should we hire aides? Move him into Wesley with Mother? Take him to the hospital?

Then Chris says, in that way a perfect stranger can size up your situation when you can't, "Have you asked him what he wants?"

The next day, we ask.

After a pause, my father answers with that quiet certainty of his: "I want to go to the hospital."

I had no idea he'd go from Brenda's to the hospital. Why did I ask Brenda to take him back that last time? If only I'd known how short this part would be. I have a crazy impulse to move him quickly to my house, then to the hospital. But of course, not possible.

Meanwhile, Brenda and Chris, who both love to cook, are having a New Year's Eve dinner at Brenda's. Naturally, Henry and I are invited, but I'm totally left out of the planning. It's as though I don't exist. The two of them fill the hours with recipe talk. Brenda's marinated veal chops. Chris's green peas and Boursin cheese. Brenda's chocolate sheet cake. Chris's something with apples.

The morning before New Year's Eve, Henry and I are making up the bed. He's on one side; I'm on the other. Each of us tugs the top sheet to make it even. Now there's too much on my side. He pulls. Too much on his. I pull—and start crying. It all feels incredibly hopeless. Too many shifts taking place. The bed, the covers, Mother, Daddy, Donald's marriage ending, Brenda.

"I don't want to go New Year's Eve," I sob. "Brenda and I . . . Our Thanksgiving Day truce was temporary. . . . We're in an awful place. . . . The whole thing will be so strained. . . . I don't really know Chris. . . . It feels as though Brenda and I are competing for her." If Donald can't be the judge, we'll just give Chris the title. Isn't she the next best thing? Brenda is definitely working hard to win her over. (We don't know at this point that Donald and Chris's romance will end before spring.) The idea of a dinner together makes my teeth hurt.

"Just call and say we're not coming," Henry says.

I love this about him. He can take a situation and, as if he's turning it over and over in the palm of his hand, see every facet. Plus, he's always looking out for me. I hadn't even thought of refusing the invitation. In the way that he's so clear-eyed, my husband is like my father.

I don't remember Brenda's reaction to my backing out. Donald tried to talk me into coming, and when I held fast, he let me know he didn't understand. *It's New Year's Eve. We should all be together.* It was hard for me to stand my ground.

26

Instead of celebrating New Year's Eve with my sister and brother, Henry and I push open the door to my father's hospital room.

This morning, the doctor changed his pain medication. My father told me on the phone that he's hurting, even with the new prescription.

I kiss his stubbly cheek, he tells me he's still in pain, I buzz the nurses' station.

"Yes?" A static-y voice.

"Could a nurse come to my father's room?" I say.

The reception clears. "Sure."

No one appears. Twenty minutes go by. Maybe more.

I buzz again.

"My father's in pain," I say, harsher than I mean to sound.

Minutes later, a nurse with wide hips pushes her way into the room and then stands there, looking at me, definitely not pleased. *Another annoying family member*, she's thinking.

"I just gave him his medicine," she says. "Right before you came. It'll take effect soon."

"How long do you think that'll be?" I ask.

"If he's not feeling better in an hour, let me know."

"An hour?" As though she said a month. "It doesn't seem like this new medication is working."

Henry catches my elbow. He knows my hospital personality.

The nurse turns to leave. "Listen," she says, now almost out in the hall, "I understand your concern, but I've got a lot of other patients on the floor to take care of, and we're short staffed. It's a holiday, you know. Let's give this medicine a chance to work."

Why does she have to say "medicine"? Is it codeine? Morphine? Why can't she treat us like adults and call the medication by name?

Henry walks over to my father. "Dad," he says quietly, "how about getting up for a while, maybe sit in the chair and give your back a rest? They don't want you staying in bed."

Henry helps him sit up and swing his legs over the side. I lie across the foot of the bed. My father's legs are the legs of an old man: hairless, yellowish, like beached fish, especially right above his ankles where tight dress socks over the years have worn them to a shine.

Slowly, Henry walks my father to the chair in the corner. He pulls up a chair for himself, next to my father. We stay like this for maybe a half-hour. My father tells about the awful supper he had at 4:30 and is beginning to tell us something about the nurse. In the middle of his sentence, though, he stops and stares at the dense shadows out the window.

"I see shapes," he says, his voice now dreamy and distant, cottony.

"What kind of shapes?" I ask.

"See? There. Your mother." He raises his eyebrows and smiles. "Hey, darlin'!" he says brightly, as though he's sitting at the breakfast-room table back on Eden Terrace, eating a bowl of cornflakes and sliced banana, and my mother has just walked in.

Then, even more brightly—almost twinkly—he says, "Look! She's playing the piano! She's playing 'Humoresque.' She has on her white pumps and blue dress, the one with all the lace at the hem. What a stunning woman she is, your mother. . . ."

I strain to see her in the darkness.

Then, as suddenly as my mother appeared, I can tell by the slope of my father's shoulders, she's gone.

He closes his eyes. Is he going to cry?

After a few seconds, Henry asks him, "Want to go to bed?"

My father opens his eyes, turns toward Henry, and grins wryly. "Not tonight, dear. I have a headache."

I'm thirty-eight years old, and this is the first off-color joke I've ever heard from my father. Henry and I begin to laugh. Then my father starts laughing, a strong and healthy laugh. Soon we're laughing and crying—all three of us—big, heaping, messy sobs. We're laughing and crying so hard we can't stop.

The nurse comes in, her hips filling the doorway again. She's carrying a Styrofoam pitcher of ice, paper cups, and a bouquet of those flexible straws. She looks surprised, then disapproving. *The daughter complains her father's in pain, and the next minute the old guy is laughing so hard he's crying?* Yes, she's definitely disapproving. But for the life of us, we can't stop. We laugh as though my father said the funniest thing in the world. We cry as though he said the saddest thing in the world.

The next morning, New Year's Day, Donald and Chris fly back to New York. My father slips into a coma.

January 2 and January 3 (my parents' forty-eighth anniversary): coma.

Early the morning of January 4, 1980, a nurse calls to say we should come to the hospital as soon as possible. His breathing has slowed and is labored.

Brenda and Chuck, Henry and I wreathe his bed. We watch him take a breath, and then we wait for the next one. His breathing keeps time with the clock on the wall. Every now and then, there's a pause between breaths, and we lean toward him, not knowing whether to hope for another breath, or the opposite. He lies on his side, hands curled in and tucked under his chin, knees drawn up. The nurse says someone should remove his ring. Since I'm on that side of the bed, I slide his ring off, surprised at how loose it is, surprised at how cold the marblelike gemstone feels, its blue veins.

By that afternoon, nothing has changed. We leave the room for a quick lunch downstairs in the cafeteria. Brenda and I, Henry and Chuck talk around Brenda's and my difficulties. Everyone is too sad to be mad.

While we're eating our grilled cheese sandwiches, our father takes his last breath.

27

Mother's death is something that seems impossible to attain. All around me, people who want to live more than anything are dying. They're having car wrecks and heart attacks, getting cancer; even their children are being killed in freak accidents, falling from sliding boards, choking on meat. It's been six years since Mother's diagnosis, a little over a year since my father's death. I read obituaries in the paper and covet those deaths for her. But she seems immune to dying.

I write fifty pages of a novel about a young woman whose mother is in the final stages of Alzheimer's. The daughter can't bear to see her mother suffer—just visiting her is like a reach into darkness—so she decides to put an end to the mother's suffering by killing her. Death will not only free the mother; it will allow the daughter to finally find the dividing line between the two of them.

Mother has no idea whether I come to see her or not. Brenda and I, still apart, do not coordinate our visits. We don't coordinate anything. The only time we talk is when we have to make a decision about Mother or the nursing home. I feel so responsible for Mother, though, that I act as if it's up to me—and only me—

to make sure the nurses on her floor know her family is checking in often, keeping watch. I'm sure I sound officious when I report back to Brenda.

One Saturday morning, Henry and I are at Mike's basketball game, sitting high in the stands with the other parents, clapping when our team runs onto the court, standing and cheering when one of our boys scores. I'm next to a physician, whose son is on the team. I don't know him well, although I've seen him at games; I know his wife better.

I turn to him and ask, "How can you kill a person without anyone finding out? I mean, isn't there a way to inject something in a person's vein that would go undetected? Like in the ankle?" I neglect to mention I'm asking this because of my novel.

Eyes straight ahead, not turning even a half-inch toward me, he says, "Judy, we're trained to save lives, not end them."

I abandon the novel. Stick with poetry.

My mother's life does not end. Other than Alzheimer's, she's healthy.

I could never have imagined that one day I would find myself longing for her death.

Around dinnertime, September 26, 1981, a nurse on Mother's floor calls to say she's running a fever.

"Should I come?" I ask. Nurses have called to give this sort of report many times during the two years Mother has been at Wesley. It always turns out to be nothing.

"No, no. No need to rush out here," she says. "We've started her on an antibiotic, and she's already better."

Why would they give an Alzheimer's patient antibiotics?

The next morning, in a condo clubhouse, five women and I are leading an all-day workshop. The workshop, called a Sampler, covers poetry, journal writing, yoga, and personal organizing. My part of the program is to lead a poetry-writing exercise. We haven't started yet; we're meeting the twenty or thirty participants, getting them registered, handing out nametags.

In the kitchen, a phone rings.

Someone picks up.

"Judy, it's for you."

I move toward the kitchen, the receiver is handed to me, I hear Judy Pera's voice. I've known Judy for years; ours is a long and comforting history.

She tells me she just spoke with Brenda. A nurse had tried to reach me, then dialed Brenda. Brenda called Judy Pera to ask if she knew where I was. Because I'd told Judy about the workshop, she was able to find me.

The next words I hear: "Jude, your mom died."

That sentence will ring in my ears for years. I can replicate the exact tone: *Juuude* (drawn out like a question), *your* (goes up on the scale) *mom* (higher) *died* (lower).

She dies on September 27, 1981, my father's birthday. Mattie tells me, "Mr. Bennie came for Mrs. Peggy. He said, *It's my birthday. Come on, it's time for me and you to go.*"

My parents are spared each other's death. My father is spared because he died first. Mother is spared because she was gone long before either of them died. I can almost hear my mother—that same belief that outcomes are always better than anyone could have hoped for—saying, "Aren't we lucky? Neither of us had to go through grieving for the other!"

28

The exact moment is unclear when Brenda and I mend the rift that started with our children going to camp, that was deepened by my asking her to take our father back, that was intensified by her situation with her oldest son, made irresolvable by something complex and delicate—two sisters who just could not figure out a way to get back together.

Around the time of Mother's death, but before the funeral, I receive the following letter from Brenda:

Dear Judy,

I think it will be easier for me to write some of my thoughts about what's been going on.

I get the feeling you want nothing more to do with me. I know that you feel hurt. Well, I am really very, very sorry for any and all of the things that I've done and said. I have a terrible temper—I always have had if you'll remember back—and I probably always will. Just remember one thing—nothing I have done was ever done with the intention of hurting you. I get mad and I do things in the heat of the moment. I am also moody, impatient, and irritable. But not on purpose. I try very hard to control these things—you just don't know how hard I try and how **very badly** I want to get along with you. I'm willing to do and try **anything** to work things out with you.

You know, a lot of water has gone under the bridge. There have been a lot of hurts—and I mean a lot—on my side, too. There have been things that have happened that have cut me deeply, but I don't see any point in opening up old wounds and rehashing them with each of us defending ourselves. What's done is done. We have very different personalities and philosophies of life, and I guess it's understandable that we would hurt each other. The point is—where do we go from here? There must be some way that we can work these things out.

The important thing is this—we're sisters—I care about you! I love you and want more than anything to get along with you. I'll try anything and do anything I can possibly do to make the situation better between us. If I only knew **what** to do, I'd do it.

Love,

Brenda

Immediately, I call her, eager for—and expecting—resolution. But not long into the conversation, her tone of voice lets me know she's miffed again. What prompted her to write the letter, what prompted this renewed frustration, how I respond, what happens next—all that will be lost to me in the pall that is cast over everything by the loss of our last parent.

She and I plan the funeral, greet and thank and hug friends

and relatives at the service, all the while barely acknowledging one another.

At the burial, though, we stand side by side, the traditional torn black ribbons of mourning pinned to our dark dresses, the earth so wet and soft our heels sink if we stand in one place too long. As the rabbi chants the Mourner's Kaddish, we step closer to one another. Her upper arm brushes my shoulder. Our heads nod a little, as though we're agreeing we both simply wanted too much. We watch the first shovels of dirt land on the casket, the sound like heavy, heavy rain, a pounding unlike the sound the leaves make, blowing softly around us, signaling a new season and our silent pact that we *will* find a way to get along.

We won't ever discuss what happened between us. Brenda and I are just not capable. We can be like a car stuck in mud. Press on the gas, press, press, the rear wheels spin, and all we've done is dig in deeper. Instead, we'll be careful with one another. If I sense a problem arising, I'll retreat, let time pass, start fresh. She'll do the same. Neither of us wants to enter that off-limits zone again.

Three weeks after Mother's funeral, I turn forty. Mother always told Brenda and me that the forties are the best years of a woman's life. I've looked forward to them for as long as I can remember, which I suppose is a little odd—a girl in her twenties and thirties, waiting (eager) to turn forty.

But she's right. My forties *are* good years.

I'm free from the shiver of my parents' illnesses.

And I have my sister.

We're back to long, chirpy phone conversations, family dinners at her house and mine, Sunday-night pizza out, ice cream afterward. She's copying recipes for me, a new sun-dried tomato and cream cheese appetizer, a squash casserole that's a little different from Mattie's, I'm making small jokes, she's recommending

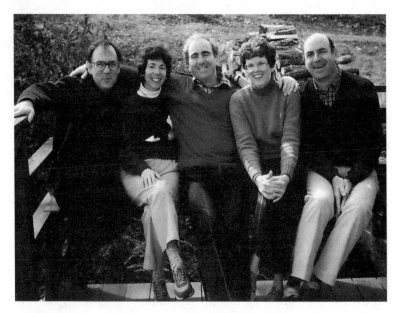

With Donald, Henry, Brenda, and Chuck, 1982

shampoos. We whisper to one another at parties, shop together
in the store. Sunday afternoons, we play Scrabble, placing each
tile so precisely, so straight and true, nothing can shake it loose.

29

Two sisters left, one set of memories:

Mother, Brenda, and I are shopping for fall clothes, 1944. My father is in the navy and soon will receive a discharge for a minor medical problem, but we don't know this yet. The three of us pass a sailor on the street. Brenda and I start singing, "Bell bottom trousers, coat of navy blue. I love a sailor and he loves me, too. . . ." Our lives could be an MGM musical, a Technicolor movie in which two sisters break into song on Main Street, bringing the family back together again.

❦

It's 1949 and my mother and father, Brenda and I are spending the last week of summer at the Ocean Forest Hotel in Myrtle Beach. The hotel is a white sandcastle of a building. On the lower level, there are a beauty salon, shoeshine stand, alteration lady, dry cleaner, gift shop. Whatever the hotel does not provide, Mother will. At night, she sprinkles talcum powder in our beds so that our skin, more and more sunburned every day, will not stick to the sheets. Brenda and I drift off to sleep in a room that smells like roses.

Our last night, there's a dinner dance in the grand ballroom. The band plays a jazzy "Humoresque," our family's favorite song, and our parents get up to dance. Brenda and I weave through the tables and chairs, closer to the dance floor. Together, we sway in time to the music. Mother is wearing a lipsticky-red and white print sundress, the gathered skirt starched stiff. In her hair, over each ear, a tortoise-shell comb, one holding a white gardenia. Her arms are tanned and her nails shaped and polished. Even though she's wearing high heels, she dances on her tiptoes. I love the way she tilts herself up to our father, the way he takes over. He's wearing his good summer suit, a brown gabardine, and brown and

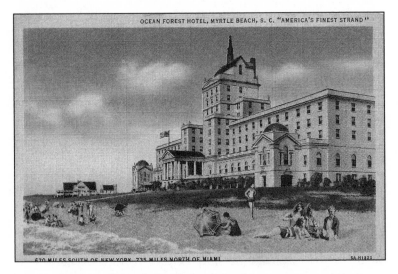

Ocean Forest Hotel, Myrtle Beach, South Carolina, 1940s

white wingtips. Brenda and I are dressed alike in buttery pink sleeveless dresses. Of course, I love dressing like Brenda; she does not love dressing like me. The crystal chandeliers have so many glimmering prisms it looks as if the moon is cracking into pieces and falling over our bare arms. Brenda and I reach out, pretend we're grabbing confetti.

♣

Mother, Brenda, and I are visiting Mrs. Landauer, 1950. Mrs. Landauer is at least twenty years older than our mother, but Mother likes visiting old people. At least that's what Brenda and I think. Mrs. Landauer's name is Salome—in private, Brenda and I call her Salami. She and her husband live in an old white house on College Avenue. They smell mothbally, like their house.

Mother sits on one faded sofa in the living room, Mrs. Landauer on the other. Brenda finds a rickety chair in the corner and opens her Nancy Drew mystery. I've brought a deck of cards and lie on my stomach on the Oriental rug. I shuffle the cards and lay them out for Solitaire. Mother and Mrs. Landauer are talking, but mostly Mrs. Landauer talks and Mother listens. During the long afternoon, Mrs. Landauer brings Brenda and me lemonade, and she and Mother have iced tea. Brenda reads. I play my game, scratching the front of my legs when the rug, with its restless pattern, gets itchy.

From the start, this game is different from others I've played. I turn over cards and instantly find places for them. There goes the jack of spades. The two of clubs. Queen of hearts.

Finally, miraculously, I'm down to one card.

And then, I find a spot for that card. All cards face up. I'm out! I've actually won a game of Solitaire! My first ever!

But I'm so shy I stay here on the rug, under the dark oil

painting of Mrs. Landauer when she was a girl, and I don't say a word. I'm so excited I can hardly stand it. Still, I don't make a sound.

⚜

I'm in nursery school, 1945. During a rare brave moment, tell the teacher, Mrs. Forsythe—we call her Mrs. So Forth—I have a song I want to sing for the class.

"Good, Judy," she says in her floral voice. "That'll be real nice." Her exact words.

She then quiets everyone, tells them I'm going to sing, and motions me to the front of the room.

I look at all those expectant faces. They begin blurring in and out of focus. *Why in the world am I doing this? What was I thinking?*

I become so paralyzed with fear I end up mouthing the entire song. The amazing thing is that because Mrs. Forsythe makes a point of gazing at me as though she can actually hear words, as though music is filling the room, my classmates sit as still and polite and attentive as little diplomats.

Years pass and I'm married, living in Charlotte. Mother and I are out for lunch in Rock Hill and run into Mrs. Forsythe. She's in her nineties, but her mind is sharp. The first thing she says is, "Judy, dear, I'll never forget the day you sang an entire song to the class without making a sound."

Mrs. Forsythe is like my mother. They're so sympathetic, I could communicate with them through my skin.

⚜

Our father, Brenda, and I are all three lying in Brenda's bed, the shade on the lamp between our beds casting a golden circle. Our father is reading aloud to us, our favorite, a Mrs. Piggle-Wiggle book. Mrs. Piggle-Wiggle is a pudgy, ageless woman who's called upon by parents to cure their children's bad habits. She has a selfishness cure, a never-want-to-go-to-bedder's cure, a thought-you-saider's cure. Our father's voice is so soft and southern, it's almost fragrant. Those thick, round vowels. Brenda and I lean in to him from both sides.

❧

Family stories grow to be bigger than the experiences themselves. They become home to us, tell us who we are, who we want to be. Over the years, they take on more and more embellishments and adornments until they eclipse the actual memories. They *become* our past—just as a snapshot will, at first, enhance a memory, then replace it.

I'm thinking of lines I read years ago in a poem, "Three Score and Five," by Marion Cannon. The narrator in the poem goes to the cemetery where her parents are buried. She writes, "I wept because there's no one living now who can remember the child I was."

I'm lucky, though. Brenda remembers. It's what sisters do.

30

It's late spring 1995, fourteen years since Mother died, a year since Donald moved to Charlotte. For months, he wondered aloud, "What would it be like if I moved back down south?" Then he sold his New York ad agency to a London firm, turned his interest in wine into a business in London, where he lived briefly, and brought his wine business—and himself (he's single)—to Charlotte. He bought a townhouse five minutes down Carmel Road from Brenda and Chuck, fifteen minutes from Henry and me. Brenda and I are glad to have him in our orbit. We're finding that we're actually good at this—the three of us joining forces. At the same time, even with the swell of camaraderie among us, there's still that almost-exclusive bond between my sister and me.

I'm sitting at my kitchen table, talking to her on the phone. Our conversation is slow and easy, rambling. She says she never understood why she's always been drawn to gardens with white-

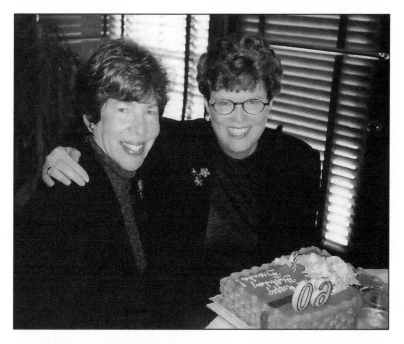

With Brenda on her 60th birthday, 1999

painted rocks along the borders—until today, when she was cleaning out a drawer and came across a black-and-white snapshot of the two of us. We're in the slatted-wood swing in the yard on Eden Terrace. She thinks she's maybe eleven, which means I'm eight. She describes the picture: We've stopped playing long enough to pose for the camera. We're wearing cotton sundresses and sandals, and both of us have barrettes in our hair. Behind us are Mother's flower beds—and the white-painted rocks that line them.

I remember when Mother had those rocks put into place, how she was afraid they'd be a breeding ground for snakes and we weren't allowed to play near them. Still, she liked their neat definition and kept them there.

After Brenda and I hang up, I stay at the table, thinking about my own garden and the changes I'll make before the summer heat sets in. I'll plant a gardenia bush next to the screened porch, shape the ivy around the yews. But then my mother's garden comes clear in my mind, the way it was when we were growing up.

Spring at our house meant red tulips circling the oak in the front yard. Spring meant forsythia blooms, yellow as stars. It was in spring when my sister and I poured bottles of Mercurochrome around the roots of the dogwood trees, determined to turn the white flowers pink.

In summer, Mother would make her way around the beds on her knees, weeding, her hands flying like small birds. She'd leave little piles of crabgrass and wild onions to collect later. I watched from the den window, all the windows and doors on the back of the house open. Every now and then, she'd stand, fan away the gnats that stuck to her face. Then she'd drag the hose across the lawn, wave it over her flowers like a wand, turning the water into an arc that crossed itself over and over. To reach the privet hedge in the back, she blocked half the flow with her fingers.

Like Mother, Brenda is a natural gardener.

When Brenda was ten, she built a fishpond in the yard. She dug the hole, mixed and poured and shaped the concrete herself. City workers had been repairing a sidewalk up the street, and Brenda had lugged home a discarded, half-empty bag of cement mix.

Newly married, Brenda planted tomatoes, squash, and cucumbers outside her kitchen door. Always, she had flowers.

Now her beds are filled with hydrangeas, roses, perennials. They climb posts, spill onto the lawn.

My own history with gardening is different. The only time I got dirt under my fingernails was when I stuffed plastic geraniums in a window box that came with the duplex Henry and

I rented when Laurie was born. Even after we moved into the split-level and Mike was born, gardening wasn't high on my list. I planted one red azalea.

Then we moved again, into a newly built house (Henry's choice) in an old neighborhood (my choice). I visited a daylily farm and bought pale peach and cream-colored daylilies. I planted tulip bulbs. Then coneflowers and phlox. I bought good pruning shears, started reading about soil amendment. Now I have shade beds and sun beds, a stone path, an arbor in the back corner. I've trained variegated ivy to twist around its angles.

Brenda and I love to talk gardening. It's a perfect subject for us—for three reasons:

One. She's more knowledgeable than I. She has even completed a master-gardening course. Every spring, I ask her the same question: "Now *when* do I prune my hydrangeas? Before they bloom or after?" Every spring, she explains that you prune Mophead, Lacecap, and Oakleaf before August, PeeGee and Limelight anytime but summer, Annabelle anytime but spring. This is a pattern that works well for us: She's the older sister who knows. I'm the younger sister who wants to know.

Two. Gardening is a subject that's *out there*, not in close. We can explore it together without fear of getting in out of our depth.

Three. Acknowledging that gardening is Mother's *and* Brenda's province wears the edges off those old divides, our usual teams. Of course, they'll never be erased completely. But maybe my sister and I can begin to learn who we are. On our own. Outside the context of our parents.

Every September, Brenda and I drive all over town together searching for the combination of pansies we've each dreamed up. I tell her what I'm looking for so she can help me find it. She tells me, and I help her. Pastel yellow and pastel blue. Purple, lavender,

and white. Burgundy and whatever there is to go with that.
We take gardening classes together.

She shares her Becky daisies with me; I share my creeping
Jenny with her.

I wish Mother could see us making our way around our yards
on our knees, weeding. I wish she could stand beside us on a hot
July day and feel the spray from the garden hose, know this extraordinary thing she's passed down to both of us, see us aim for
the back hedge, turning the water into an arc that crosses itself
over and over.

31

I write the first draft of my novel, *The Slow Way Back*, in three months, then spend the next three years revising. The two main characters, Mickey and Thea, are of course based on Brenda and me. All the while I'm writing and rewriting, I worry that she'll take offense at what I've done. In fact, I wait until I know the book will be published before I give her a copy. If it's never published, why put the two of us through turmoil? Well, why put me through turmoil?

The day I sign the contract with the publisher, I give a copy of the manuscript to Brenda.

Early the next morning, she calls. She's been up all night reading.

I can feel my heart hammering. Like a motor trying to catch. I know she could hate what I've written. What right do I have to publish a book that's essentially a fictional account of the two of us?

But she doesn't hate it. She's complimentary. She likes the

story, and the writing. She especially likes the character based on her—strong, capable, decisive Mickey.

When the book is published in 1999, my publisher throws a party for me at a museum in Charlotte. I give a talk, read from the book, sign copies. Brenda has brought a friend to the event, and the friend is standing in line, along with others, waiting for me to autograph her book. Brenda, laughing good-naturedly, brings her friend's book to the table to show me that she, Brenda, has already signed it. The name she used in her inscription: *Mickey.*

This is the novel in which each sister discovers a lump in her breast, but they face different results.

While there is plenty in my novel for Brenda to object to, the biggest risk is allowing the character based on her to die of recurring cancer. Now it's obvious to me that I was unconsciously preparing myself for the grief of losing my sister. Which of course is a totally useless dress rehearsal. You can't practice death.

As I was writing the scene, I kept trying to put on brakes, to keep Mickey from dying. *No. Stop. Let's have a happier ending.* But my fingers continued typing. When I finished, my hands moved of their own accord to my face. My cheeks were wet with tears. I had no idea that the whole time I was writing, I'd been sobbing.

Here's that passage:

> *In the hospital again. Terrible, half-torn sounds of coughing, the choking, gasping. A glass by the bed to hold sputum.*
>
> *The snaky tubes. Harder for her to breathe now. Sleeping most of the time.*
>
> *Coma. The machines, their insistent sighs.*
>
> *The winter sky out the window lavender, like the beginning of a bruise.*

And then one sister peacefully, irrevocably disentangling herself from the other. Breaking free.

All their lives Mickey had protected her. Spoken for her. Thought for her. Thea had studied Mickey's face to find out if she approved of her. Studied Mickey's face to find out if Thea approved of Thea. All their lives Thea had clung to her.

Now, for the first time, she could not follow.

She climbed into the hospital bed to lie beside her, pulled the blanket, stubbled after so many hospital launderings, over both of them, tucking it under their chins like a muffler.

Thea's body was an outline of her sister's, their fingers scalloped.

BrendaandJudy.

32

On a family road trip to Miami Beach, winter of 1953, in our box of an Oldsmobile, our parents were pointing out the sights. "Look! Out this window! Palm trees! Coconuts!"

But the two of us (fifteen and twelve) were deep in the back seat, our hair falling around our faces. We were busy flipping the pages of movie magazines, *Photoplay*, *Modern Screen*, swapping them back and forth. Our parents thought we were shutting out everything good the state of Florida had to offer. Brenda and I paid them no mind. We could've been floating away on disks of stardom.

When we arrived in Miami Beach, my father waited at the curb while Mother, Brenda, and I checked out the pastel lobbies and available rooms in every hotel on Collins Avenue. We debat-

ed (the Saxony? Sherry Frontenac? Delmonico?), finally decided
on the Martinique.

In our room, which adjoined our parents', Brenda slid open
the glass doors to step out onto the balcony; she stood there, her
hair lifting in the ocean breeze. Quickly, I slid the doors shut,
turned the lock, scribbled one word on a sheet of hotel stationery,
and held it up to the glass. "JUMP!" it said. We were so giddy
about all that glamour, about having our own room, about wearing shorts and halters in January, anything either of us did would
have cracked the other up. We laughed so hard at my joke we had
to hold our sides.

🪷

December 2001. Brenda has been having stomach pains. At
times, mild. At times, not so mild. "Mostly," she tells me, "they're
something I can live with."

Initially, the internist checked her, said she was okay. Then
her pains worsened. The internist was puzzled. He sent her to a
gastroenterologist, who ordered blood work and an MRI. Something's definitely wrong, the gastroenterologist said. He knows
she had breast cancer in 1992, so he's being hypervigilant. But
then: she's all right; everything's fine. The back-and-forthing—
she's not fine, she is fine—the whole month. Brenda's belief is that
it's nothing. As though it's a storm the weather people on TV
are hyping as severe, and we pull out our flashlights, stock up on
bread and milk, then are relieved to see out the window only a
slight breeze rustling the air.

She's still working. Harder than ever. She now runs a large
mail-order gift-basket company called Gifts To Go. Chuck closed
our father's two stores in Rock Hill and is working with Brenda.
Their busy season, September through Christmas, just ended.

She started the company, doing everything herself—from conceiving the idea to assembling the baskets to marketing. In the beginning, she made bows—hundreds of them—at night while she and Chuck watched TV. Then she filled baskets (special ones with unusual textures and shapes) with shortbread, cheese straws, jams, pound cakes. Not just ordinary shortbread, cheese straws, jams, and pound cakes. Whatever she placed in those baskets was the best she could find. By the time she shrink-wrapped and decorated a basket with ribbons and bows, there was a rightness to it, a shimmering, as though she'd pumped light in. Brenda has an artist's eye *and* remarkable business acumen *and* the perseverance to see a project through. Every business she creates is successful. She's always been a person full of reach.

❧

Brenda and I, Laura and Helen O'Neal (who lived behind us), and the Dickerts (all six children, next door on Eden Terrace) put on shows for the rest of the neighborhood in the empty henhouse in the Dickerts' backyard. The stage was a narrow wooden platform above an open space where the audience sat. The door through which the actors entered and exited hung on one hinge.

Our most memorable performance: Brenda had pushed baking potatoes up her sleeves to look like muscles. She arched one eyebrow, flexed those muscles, shouted with what she thought was a Russian or maybe Bulgarian accent, "Me strong!"

Laura, wearing somebody's old glasses, pointed to her head, declared, "Me smart!"

I slumped, jutted my chin out as though it was all I knew to do, and murmured pathetically, "I've been sick."

We brought down the house. Brenda's muscles alone were worth the price of admission.

❧

January 2, 2002. Brenda sees the gastroenterologist for a follow-up. He's concerned and orders additional blood work and testing. This news makes my arms cold, the way a chill can set in before the heat comes on in the house.

❧

Tonight, January 6, 2002, Henry and I have dinner at Brenda and Chuck's. (They built a new house not long ago, on the lot next to their old house.) For appetizers, Brenda serves a sampling of dips—tapenade, salsa, bean dip. "They're new products for my gift baskets," she says, sitting beside me on the loveseat. Chuck is in the black leather recliner (not a La-Z-Boy, but a Stickley-style from Restoration Hardware). He's what you'd call strapping, tall and muscular. His most commented-upon feature is his nearly bald head, which gives him a striking, urbane appearance. He started losing his hair in his twenties. Henry is on the other loveseat. He's spooning bean dip onto a cracker, shaping it with a little hors d'oeuvre knife. "They're low fat," Brenda says. "I wanted to see what y'all think."

"Well, that gives me an idea for your next business!" I say. Brenda finds great turtlenecks at Costco, jewelry at the flea market, low-fat foods nobody else has heard of. "You could start a newsletter," I say. "*Brenda's Hot Tips!*"

She laughs. "Oh, Judy, you're always coming up with businesses for me! I couldn't do that. No way. You're right, I do know what I like. But I'm not interested in everybody else doing what I'm doing."

Tonight is an inadvertent celebration. Just before we arrived, Brenda heard from the doctor about her tests. They did not show anything. She's optimistic, so the three of us are, too. We make a cozy half-circle around the flames in the fireplace. We could put our hands around this whole evening and press it, tight.

❧

January 19, 2002. I drive to Winston-Salem to visit my cousin Debbie (Aunt Katie's daughter). This morning, Brenda will hear the results of her latest tests. Her digestive problems have worsened—the pain, at times, thick.

After I park my car in Debbie's driveway and I'm admiring the pansies, a crush of purple on both sides of the front steps, my cell phone rings.

It's Brenda. Her voice is matter-of-fact: "I have cancer of the bile duct." Then, not so matter-of-fact: "I just can't believe it! This is so, so hard to take in!" Matter-of-fact again: "The prognosis is about the same as it is for pancreatic cancer. Not good. Not good at all." The doctor is now convinced. "I'm dealing with it, though. Just like I dealt with breast cancer," she says. "I don't like it, but it is what it is."

An hour from now, I won't remember what I said or how the rest of the conversation went. I said something. She said something. We talked and talked. I *will* remember that the morning sun—a winter sun at that—was suddenly burning sharp and hot.

❧

February 15, 2002. Brenda now knows what is next for her: Whipple surgery. The word sounds whimsical, but it's actually the name of a complicated and serious operation that can take as long as eight hours. The surgeon will remove her gall bladder and duodenum, a portion of her pancreas and bile duct. Some of her stomach may also have to be removed. Then what remains of the intestinal tract will have to be reconnected. She's been told that her digestive system will never be the same. She may need to take pancreatic enzymes to help her absorb food. She could develop diabetes. It's a long and painful recuperation. I ache for what she's about to endure.

❦

March 2002. Brenda has her surgery, and it takes the full eight hours. Chuck, their sons, Henry and I cluster in the family waiting area. We talk, try to read, leave the room and circle the halls, talk more, pick up the same leathery-with-use magazines, circle again.

After the surgery, she is *so* sick. In fact, she's the same degree of sick every day—and remains in the hospital—for twenty-eight days. No change, not a glint of improvement. She can't take even a drop of water. She has an IV in her arm, a tube up her nose, a surgical drain from her abdomen, a catheter, a morphine pump. Pain, fever, dizziness, sweats, chills, grey bile vomit—until one day, it's as if we stumble into the presence of a miracle, and she is suddenly better.

The very next morning, Chuck takes her home.

33

It's March 2004, two years after Brenda's Whipple surgery. Although she's thin and has digestive problems from the surgery, she's regained much of her strength and is playing duplicate bridge again, gardening, and, since she and Chuck have both retired, they're traveling all over the country and Europe. She's tough; very little keeps my sister down.

I decide it's time to give manuscripts of my second novel, *Early Leaving*, to Brenda and to Donald. It tells the story of an overprotective mother whose son, a graduating high-school senior, top scholar, and star athlete, commits murder. The plot has nothing at all to do with my sister and me. During the three years I was writing and revising, Brenda told me more than once that she and Chuck were eager to read it. But, as with my first novel, I've waited until publication is a sure thing. I'm happy to stay as long as possible in that wordless space—before what I've written will be read, before my sister can react to it.

The day after I give Brenda and Donald copies of my manuscript, Donald calls. He's finished reading, and it's clear from the things he says that he's rooting for me. His words feel like seeds of light.

It takes Brenda longer. After several weeks, she calls to discuss the book. But as we talk, she seems to be moving farther and farther away from me. In the beginning, she's in her house in South Charlotte and I'm ten minutes away, in my house. By the middle of the conversation, she could be in South Dakota—that's how distant she sounds.

"I finished your book last week . . . but didn't have a chance to call till now because we had company over the weekend." Then she says, somewhat ruefully, "It was . . . good. Your book was, uh . . . real good." Every word is measured. A frozen politeness. As though she can't begin to say what she's really thinking.

"Thank you," I say. "Thanks."

Then there's almost a museum silence.

What can I say next? "I appreciate your reading it."

"Well . . . I found it . . . interesting," she says. "Yeah, it was interesting."

Something is changing color and shape, and I can't stop it.

I'm sitting in my office; Henry is in his. Since he retired in 2000, only a door separates his office (a spare bedroom) from mine (the upstairs landing). I push back from my desk to open the door, hit *Speaker* so he can hear what's being said. I don't trust myself to view this conversation with any objectivity. I want Henry, when it's over, to help me understand what just occurred.

"Yeah?" I say. Back to my desk.

"Yeah," Brenda says.

What are we saying yeah to?

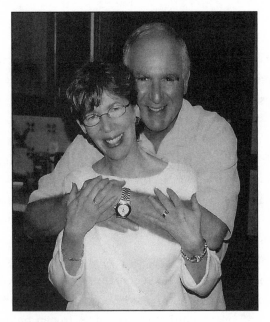

With Henry, 2004

Pause.

"It was interesting . . . ," she says again.

Longer pause.

". . . the way you used the names of your childhood friends for minor characters."

"Oh," I say, "I did that because Billy Watson kept kidding me, asking when I was going to write a book about him. So I just combined the first names of some of my Rock Hill friends with the last names of other Rock Hill friends and used those for my characters."

I want to sound loose and natural, but I'm sure that trying to set upright whatever has been tipped is changing my voice in a way that isn't helping.

Silence.

"You probably recognized some of the details I took from real life," I suggest.

"Like what?"

I get up from my desk and stand in the doorway to Henry's office. I search his face. He cocks his head to let me know he, too, finds her reaction puzzling.

"Well, the details from our childhood," I say. "I mean, yours and mine. And from Laurie and Mike's."

"Hmm. I don't know. Like what?"

"Well, let me think." Maybe I should stay away from memories that involve her. "The time Mike got bitten in the face by a dog."

"I wouldn't really remember that." Vague has now turned to negative. How can she not remember one of the scariest things that ever happened to any of our children? I remember everything significant that happened to her children. Of course she remembers.

Then she tells me the prison scene was well done. (Negative turns to positive.) She also liked the ending. She thought that was beautiful. But there are a couple of things she had trouble with, she says, and she names those: There should have been some hint of problems along the way before the teenager in the book commits murder. That seemed sudden and implausible. And why didn't I follow up on the temper tantrums he had as a child? How could they just disappear when he's older? That would never happen in real life.

Positive has turned to critical.

"But you know," she says, "I'm not really a critic, and I'm probably wrong, and anyway, I read it in such a hurry, I probably missed a lot."

Vague to negative to positive to critical, finally landing on indifferent.

34

Henry's opinion: "I think the two of you were back into your big sister/little sister thing. You, seeking her approval. Brenda, withholding it. What I don't understand is why she couldn't just give it."

I don't like his opinion. Well, actually—this minute—I don't like admitting I need her approval. Of course, all those years, I would have said the same thing about myself. But now, unexpectedly, I see how pitiful it makes me sound. I decide to split hairs, find the nuanced explanation of exactly what I was looking for, let Henry know that even though I was depending on him for clarity, I disagree with his clarity.

"No," I say, snippiness built into the way I jerk one shoulder, "I don't think approval is what I was looking for. I'd say I wanted something a degree less than that. Maybe just the feeling that she's *for* me."

In other words, I get mad at the safest person around.

Days later, an icy day, the entire world under glass—my bell rings, the back door. It's Chuck, and he's holding my manuscript under his arm. He looks at me with his pale blue eyes and says that Brenda is in the car but won't be coming in because she's afraid of falling on the slippery walk. I understand; she should be careful. But then he hands over my pages and says, "Thanks. Good luck." And he's gone.

Did he read them? Does he think my book is so bad I'll *need* luck to see it through?

When I look closer at my manuscript, I see a card—Brenda's formal stationery—paper-clipped to the first page:

Dear Judy,

> *Thanks for giving me a "pre-publication peek" at "Early Leaving." With all my heart, I wish for you huge sales and literary awards! Good luck!*

Much love,

Brenda

So. She's covering her bases. She follows up her coldness on the phone by writing a note with a couple of friendly exclamation points. And let's see. What can she say that will be really nice? How about throwing in *with all my heart* and *much love?* Still, such a vigorously neutral note. It feels almost like something a publicist might write, someone whose main concerns are sales and prizes.

Is she jealous? Does my book break some unspoken pact that the older sister should be the star, the younger sister the audience?

What if it's just that she didn't like it? Isn't she entitled to not like my book? Writers can be supersensitive about family reactions to their work; why do we care so much? As a writer, I'm used to criticism; rejection is part of the job description. Why does hers bother me?

When I was ten, I entered a talent contest on the radio, singing "America, the Beautiful" with no piano, no accompaniment at all. The P.E. teacher, who played the piano for school assemblies, had offered to accompany me, but I said, "Oh, that's okay. I'll just sing." The morning of the contest, I woke with a head cold, a really bad stopped-up nose, but I was already in the-show-must-go-on mode and nothing could stop me. In fact, I was terrible. Brenda was mortified (her word) and didn't speak to me for days.

Maybe she's mortified by my book.

Now I'm thinking of all the ways it falls short. In my mind's eye, I see myself telling every person who reads it, "If you could just look inside my head, you'd see what a good writer I am. But something goes wrong between the vision I have in the beginning and the unruly words that end up on paper."

Maybe my writing a novel baffles her the same way my diaries did. Third grade through twelfth, I never missed a day, filling each page from January 1 to the last line of December 31. Brenda would start on January 1, too—we'd lie on our stomachs in our beds, hiding what we were writing with our arms—but by the end of the month, she'd moved on to something else. It annoyed her that I stayed with it. As though it was preposterous for me to be doing something she wasn't. *You're not following me, Judy. That's not all right.*

When I told Henry that I wanted Brenda to be *for* me, I could have been talking about my father. How I wanted what was important to me to be important to him. Like a magician turning a scarf into gardenias, I tried to turn both my father and Brenda into my mother. Mother's reaction always coalesced around these words: "My, my, Judy! Look what you've done!" During the years since she died, I've gotten along okay with the absence of that voice. But every now and then, when I've worked hard on something, when I have a lot at stake, I find myself wanting to hear those words again. I think I knew it wouldn't be fair to expect the "Look what you've done!" part from Brenda. But I couldn't keep myself from wanting the "My, my!"

Days after Chuck returns the manuscript, my cousin Debbie comes to town, and she, Brenda, and I go out for lunch. Suddenly, the memory of our other fight—getting our kids to camp—encloses me, like a shudder. How it escalated, one small hurt at a time, until there was big hurt on both sides. I decide I'd better try to smooth things over. Which makes me feel very magnanimous. Maybe it shows. Because Brenda is doing everything she can to let me know she's put out with me. Why is she put out with me? Shouldn't I be put out with her? She and Debbie are sitting next to each other on the banquette, and I'm across from them. All Brenda's conversation is directed toward Debbie. Brenda hardly speaks to me. She doesn't look in my direction. I could walk out of the restaurant and she wouldn't notice that the table for three just became a table for two.

35

A couple of weeks later, Brenda and I have tickets, bought months ago, for a gardening symposium in Davidson, half an hour away. This is an annual event for us, one that inspires and excites us. On the way home and for days afterward, we're full of rapturous and absorbed talk about what we've learned, how we'll start fresh in our own gardens. She's such an artist—I love seeing a landscape through her eyes. But this year, as the date and the prospect of spending time with her get closer, I feel dread.

"You don't have to go," Henry says.

"But I don't want to make this a bigger deal than it already is. If I cancel, I'm afraid it will up the ante—"

"You don't have to go, Judy. You can give yourself some time, see what you want to do about all this."

"But I'll have to say why I'm not going."

"Well, maybe that's not such a bad thing. You know, you could just tell her what's bothering you."

"But we're not good at talking things through."

Henry, strong and self-determining, has been quietly pushing me for years to free myself of my dependence on my sister. Mainly, he wants me to stand up to her, not be afraid to say what I think. It has not been an easy sell.

Finally, I make the call, tell her I know she had problems with my book and I don't expect everyone to like it—in fact, there are parts I wish I could rewrite this very minute—but her reaction hurt my feelings. It's too late for me to change anything in the book, I say, so I wasn't really looking for a critique. And, well, I'd expected something different from my sister. I tell her I don't think we should spend the day together with things the way they are between us, so I'm canceling my symposium reservation.

At one point while I'm having my say, I think, *Wow. I'm telling my big sister how I feel about something she did. Wow.*

She, obviously, is not thinking, *Wow.* She does not like what I'm saying. Her voice rising in anger, she points out that she had only one problem with the book, and that was how the son's temper tantrums could disappear so abruptly. She says she's not the only one who thought that part was not believable. Donald felt the same way and I should just ask him. (Now she's bringing in extra troops for reinforcement.)

I swallow hard. This is not going well. But what did I expect? That she would immediately say she really did like my book and doesn't know why she reacted the way she did and, gosh, she's so sorry? This conversation feels overpowering. I tell her I can't keep talking because I'm feeling too emotional, I'll call tomorrow so she can say what she wants to say.

She presses on, very aroused, wants to say what she wants to say *now.*

I do want to talk, I repeat. But can we do it later?

No, let's finish now, she says.

I promise, I'll call tomorrow. I finally say I have to hang up.

The next day, I call, but she says she doesn't want to talk to me. She's letting me know that if I wasn't willing to discuss it then (when it suited her), she's not willing to discuss it now (when it suits me).

This begins a downward spiral in which every word between us becomes proof of a lack of love, each sentence heaps on added resentment. We've entered that phase of a conflict where we're both convinced the other is twisting what actually happened.

Months pass. April, May, June.

Maybe enough time has passed that one of us could step forward, take a chance, call with the sole purpose of seeking out the other. I decide to try. I use a friendly voice. "How was your trip to Santa Fe?" I ask.

"Fine," she says. Frosty.

Now what? She's reserving her position. Letting time pass did not solve anything. And there's not going to be a summit meeting followed by a settlement.

September 2004 (six months since I gave Brenda the manuscript), my novel is published. When my first novel and my books of poetry were published, I gave copies to everyone in the family, including nephews and nieces. I think it would be terribly pointed to give books to Brenda and Chuck's sons but not to Brenda and Chuck, so I take her a copy of *Early Leaving*.

I want to appear relaxed. I'm trying to pantomime normalcy. But it's hard to breathe. And the expression on my face is, I'm sure, solemn. She and I stand just inside her door. As I hand over my book, I see the words traveling from my mouth: "Here, Brenda. I want you to have a copy. At the same time, I realize our views are different as to what went on around this."

"Very different," she says, hitting *very* like a nail.

36

Days after taking her the book:

September 24, 2004

Dear Judy,

Thank you so much for giving me a copy of your book. It is quite a thrill to actually see it in print. You have achieved so very much, and I am extremely proud of you!!

Contrary to what you seem to think, I really think the book is beautifully written, and I am sorry if I have cast any sort of shadow on the excitement and pride you must feel. I am certainly not a judge of anything—and certainly not one of anything literary, since I really know nothing of literature.

In our book club, I see myself as the least perceptive of any of us, and I am always amazed at the insights expressed by others that I never even thought of.

Let me just say, once and for all, I have no problem with your book! I do have some problems, but they are centered around trying to stay out of the bathroom and trying to not cough so much that I throw up. My only thoughts about your book have to do with amazement at what you have accomplished and pride that you are published by a major publisher and bought by people all over the country.

The only comment I made was that it seemed there should have been some hint of problems along the way before committing murder. Period! I wish I had never said it, and it is probably not even a valid comment. Certainly, it is one I wish I could take back. I do remember (even though the conversation about your book was quite some time ago) having a discussion about how moving and beautifully written the part about going to the prison the first time was. Didn't we discuss that in great detail? I really don't remember clearly, and I want to forget the whole thing. I thought we had moved forward long ago.

I hope you will accept this letter with compassion, and I don't expect any kind of answer. I am trying very hard not to have on-going stress in my life because I know it is not healthy for me, so I hope you won't read any negativity between the lines because none was intended. I simply want to live and let live in peace and harmony.

Love,

Brenda

37

Dear Brenda,

Thank you for writing me that letter. I know you were sincerely trying to put things right and at the same time, help both of us move on. I appreciate the sweet things you said.

I honestly thought I had put this behind me a long time ago. But when it came time for me to give you and Chuck a copy of my book, I realized I was still feeling sad. I know you and I remember that phone conversation differently. I think that in order for me to move on, I need to say to you what I remember. I don't expect you to see it the way I see it. I'm okay with our agreeing to disagree; I just need to tell my perspective.

I gave my manuscript to you and Chuck because you're my sister and brother-in-law, and I was eager to share with you what I'd been working on. You remember pointing out *only one fault in the book; I remember more than that. But really, the number isn't important. I wasn't giving it to you for any kind of literary criticism; it was too late for me to revise. What I wanted was someone to share excitement with, regardless of the merits or failings of the book, and when you didn't seem excited, I was disappointed and hurt. Maybe you didn't mean it that way—and maybe my wishing for that felt to you like an expectation you couldn't meet. I also want to add that Chuck's response was a part of what I reacted to. When he returned the manuscript to me, he said, "Thanks. Good luck." I couldn't tell if he'd read it or not.*

Now I've told my perspective—and I want to also tell you this:

You are a wonderful sister—and Chuck is a wonderful brother-in-law—and I love you both very much. Through the years, you've done a million thoughtful and generous things for me and shown your love in many, many ways. I also feel that the two of us, in recent years, have figured out how to have a better relationship. I don't want this one incident to overshadow all that. I also want you to know that if I could trade this book for your good health, I would do it in a second. What I pray for is for you to feel well; I hate what you have to go through and hope, with all my heart, you know that.

Much love,

Judy

38

Why is it so hard to discern what causes what?

One thing I don't yet realize: that, on some unconscious level, I must have felt this was my last chance to stand up to her. To have a voice. The little girl who stopped up her mouth with a fist in order to get her sister's attention, who sang an entire song in nursery school without making a sound, who won at Solitaire but didn't utter a word, who entered talent contest after talent contest singing and tap-dancing, never winning but continually embarrassing her sister. The little girl whose father judged whether or not her words were important enough to merit a conversation. I just wanted to have a voice, speak my mind.

I did speak my mind in small ways when we were growing up: Brenda had a habit of cracking her knuckles; I never cracked mine. My hands were so skinny it took painful force to make that snapping sound. When she'd get mad at me, she'd hold me down and crack every one of my knuckles, from my index finger down. My revenge options were limited. One that always worked: I'd march over to the piano and, with a cadenced emphasis, play the scale—C, D, E, F, G, A, B. But instead of ending on C, I purposely hit C-sharp. Then I'd casually walk away from the piano, taking great pleasure in her screams: "I can't stand when you do that!"

When she was thirteen, over five-seven, under a hundred pounds, my fighting words were, "You wear glasses and braces. What's next? A hearing aid?"

In 1952, the year Eisenhower ran against Stevenson, our parents took Brenda and me to New York to experience election night in Times Square (the same trip as the nightclub visit). I was for Eisenhower because I liked his smile; Brenda was for Stevenson because our father was for him. The most memorable moment of the trip did not take place on election night (or in the nightclub bathroom); it was when we were leaving the Imperial Theatre after the musical *Wish You Were Here*. Suddenly, our father spotted Ed Sullivan crossing the marbled floor of the lobby, just about to open the heavy doors to the outside. Brenda bolted over to get his autograph. Within minutes, hundreds of people surrounded him. I couldn't get close. Brenda emerged from the crowd, holding that precious autograph aloft. Tearful, I followed her back to our parents. Our father then steered me by the shoulders straight through to Ed Sullivan. It was like a parting of the Red Sea. After he explained what had happened, Ed Sullivan crouched down, balanced his big, square body on his heels, asked my name and where I was from, signed my little scrap of paper, looked me in the eye, and said, "Judy, if these Yankees up here give you any more trouble, you just let me know."

Into the cold, through Times Square, our breath freezing, back to the Hotel Astor, New Yorkers winging by us on all sides,

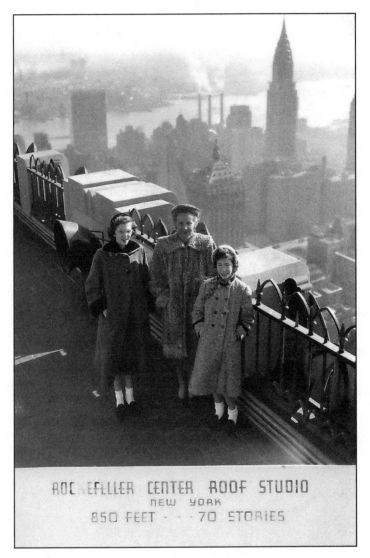

With Brenda and Mother, Rockefeller Center, New York City, 1952

into the elevator, up to our room adjoining our parents', I repeated dreamily, as though the words were set to music, " 'If these Yankees up here give you any more trouble.' . . . He said that to me . . . only me . . . not to anybody else . . . just me. . . . 'If these Yankees . . .' "

When Brenda and I were alone in our room, the door bolted, she finally grumbled, "Will you please shut up?"

Brenda's letter was an honest attempt at reconciliation. Exactly what I'd been wishing for.

But because she gave her version of what went on between us, I had to give mine. To use my father's word, I was hellbent on giving my version. That was so dumb of me. I should have let it go. I should have been grateful for the concessions she made in her letter. Grateful she cared enough to write the letter. I should have known that we all can feel one way and act another. She doesn't believe she was anything but pleased about my book. I should have accepted that, called a halt to, *But this is the way I see it, yeah but this is the way I see it.*

Most important of all, I should have realized that my sister is coping with a very grave illness, and her reaction to my book was, and is, inconsequential.

Maybe she *does* know the real Judy. The Judy who's really not so sweet. Or sensitive. Or compassionate.

39

October 20, 2004, my birthday. A wrapped package left outside my back door, with a note:

Dear Judy,

This probably seems like a strange gift, but this is a cream that I started using a few months ago, and it has made the most incredible difference. So, I thought you might like it, too, since our skin texture is so similar.

They have assured me at Nordstrom's that you can try it, and if you don't like it, you can take it back for a refund.

But I think you're going to like it! Hope so.
HAPPY BIRTHDAY!

Love,

Brenda

From the outside, this would seem a lovely way to wish a sister happy birthday—the personal gift (nothing is closer than skin!), the tentative note, even the *Hope so* squeezed in at the end of the line, obviously added later to show she wouldn't assume I'd like it just because she does.

But our tradition is to call the birthday person way ahead to make a date for lunch out—on the actual birthday. At lunch, there's a gift, along with a note that says something very loving, like how lucky we are to have gotten the other for a sister. (Mother and her sisters celebrated birthdays the same way. They even gave each other Mother's Day gifts. Brenda and I don't go that far.)

One of two things is going on:

Either Brenda is trying, once again, to reconcile, and the closest she feels she can come is to give a present and write a friendly—though several notches below loving—note in which she mentions our alikeness.

Or. She is making a statement. *Yes, I'll remember your birthday. I'll even give a present. But you know—and you know that I know—things are not right between us.*

It may sound like I'm overthinking this. But sisters are intuitively aware of each other's deepest motivations. Even unintuitive sisters know each other in a way that is beyond knowing.

40

OCTOBER 24, 2004

DEAR JUDY,

YOU LET ME KNOW SEVEN MONTHS AGO
BY HANGING UP ON ME AND BY TELLING ME
YOU WEREN'T GOING TO THE DAVIDSON SEMI-
NAR WITH ME (WHICH TO ME MEANT YOU
DIDN'T WANT ANYTHING MORE TO DO WITH
ME) THAT YOU WERE EXTREMELY ANGRY
WITH ME. I ACCEPTED THIS, WAS VERY MUCH
UPSET AND SADDENED BY IT, BUT FELT THAT
WAS YOUR PREROGATIVE. THE WHOLE THING
TOTALLY STYMIED ME.
NOW YOU HAVE EXPLAINED, IN ADDITION

TO MY CRITICISM, IT HAD TO DO WITH MY
LACK OF "EXCITEMENT" OVER YOUR BOOK.
DO YOU THINK THE FACT THAT I WAS EX-
TREMELY SICK AT THE TIME (AND, IN FACT, AS
I TOLD YOU, I COULD HARDLY HOLD THE MAN-
USCRIPT TO READ IT) COULD HAVE POSSIBLY
HAD ANYTHING TO DO WITH MY IMPROPER
RESPONSE?

I HOPE YOUR "SADNESS" IS FINALLY, AFTER
SEVEN MONTHS, ALLEVIATED.

MY SADNESS, UNFORTUNATELY, HAS IN-
CREASED. HOW A "LOVING" SISTER CAN CON-
TINUE WITH THIS IN VIEW OF WHAT WE'RE
DEALING WITH IS VERY HARD TO UNDER-
STAND. YOU AND I BOTH KNOW THE PROG-
NOSIS IS HORRIFIC FOR PANCREATIC CANCER.
DOESN'T IT SEEM ABSURD TO TAKE SEVEN
MONTHS OF WHATEVER TIME I HAVE LEFT TO
HARBOR THIS?

NOW LET'S BRING THIS THING TO A CLOSE:

YOU'RE RIGHT! **I'M** WRONG! I DID ALL THE
HORRIBLE THINGS YOU SAY I DID. AND I DID
IT WITH MEAN, EVIL, VICIOUS INTENT. I'M A
SHIT!!

THERE! NOW CAN WE LET THIS GO?

BRENDA

41

My immediate reaction:
*I WAS EXTREMELY SICK AT THE TIME (AND,
IN FACT, AS I TOLD YOU, I COULD HARDLY HOLD
THE MANUSCRIPT TO READ IT)...*
What she actually told me was that she had company that
weekend.
How sick could she have been?

My next, and enduring, reaction:
I've lived with Brenda all my life. I know her temper. I know
it's hard for her to hit the reset button. For her to venture forth
and write two "soft" notes, for her to bring a birthday gift—she
was trying the best she could. My response to that first note was
me being greedy, pushing. I should have left well enough alone.
Now I've done it. Could I have handled this whole thing any
clumsier?

42

The end of October (seven months now since she read my manuscript), Brenda and Chuck send out printed invitations for an anniversary party they're throwing for themselves—cocktails at their house, dinner at Noble's restaurant. They want to thank all their friends and family for their kindnesses during Brenda's illness. Henry and I are invited, as are our children—Laurie and husband Bob, Mike and wife Brooke.

Dear Brenda,

Thank you for your invitation. We'll definitely be there. The evening sounds really nice—forty-five years is truly something to celebrate.

In response to your letter, I'm sorry you thought I didn't want to have anything more to do with you. That was not my intention. Nor do I think you're all wrong and I'm all right. Other than that, I'm not sure saying anything else at this point will be helpful or productive. The most meaningful thing I read in your letter was that you want to move on, start over. I do, too.

Love,

Judy

43

When Henry and I arrive at Brenda and Chuck's, they both greet us, and Brenda and I actually chat. I say how beautiful the house looks. She whispers that she was worried no one would show up, since the party is the Saturday after Thanksgiving. "But look around," I say. "Everyone's here." Eighty to eighty-five people, I'm guessing. Our conversation feels natural.

In the restaurant—a private room—Brenda has placed starry votive candles everywhere and, in the center of each table, clay pots she painted mica-like gold, filled with roses. She has even handcrafted menus, listing the dinner choices.

My admiration quickly gives way to disappointment. Also bearing her personal stamp are place cards. Even before I find mine, I know this is the beginning of the hard part.

Seated at the head table (for six) are Brenda and Chuck,

Donald, Chuck's sister Doris, and Brenda's good friend and her husband. I'm the only sibling not at their table. Henry and I are at a table off to the side.

After salad and before entrées, Brenda makes her way around the room, talking with everyone. When she gets to our table, she says, "How are the folks who grew up in South Carolina doing?"

So that's the category I'm in now. Of the three couples at our table, one man grew up in Rock Hill, one woman grew up in Barnwell, and one man grew up in Fort Mill. And then, of course, there's me: just another person Brenda knows who's a native of South Carolina.

Entrée: choice of steak or salmon.

Dessert: Cake. Pie. It doesn't matter.

I keep up the chatter at our table. Henry and I know Brenda and Chuck's friends; they're always friendly to us. *Just get through the evening, Judy. You don't want to call attention to yourself by sulking or leaving early.* Laurie and Mike, seated at the kids' table with their cousins, keep coming over and patting my back. They know my sadness (and hurt and feelings of hopelessness and, yes, anger) is rising.

Chuck stands and taps his glass to quiet the room.

In a long speech, he charts his and Brenda's life together. They were college sophomores (Brenda, University of Georgia; Chuck, University of North Carolina) when they met on a blind date on New Year's Eve in Atlanta. The next morning, Brenda called home. My parents and I were on three different extensions—my father in the den, Mother at the phone table in the back hall, me upstairs on the cedar chest in the landing. "He's real good looking! And tall. And nice!" Oh, the dips and rises of Brenda's sentences. "He's from Toronto, but his family used to live in Charlotte. His parents know Uncle Easy and Aunt Fannye." I wrote everything down because, well, I always wrote everything down. Instead of a diary, though, I grabbed the pad next to the phone. For sure, Brenda had just met the man she would marry. I knew I was looking into the future. I also knew that one day she would want to recall what she had said. A year later, in December, they were married in Temple Israel in Charlotte, with a dinner afterward at the Hotel Barringer. I was her maid of honor; she gave me a gold charm for my charm bracelet, engraved, *Love, Brenda.* Just before the wedding weekend, I remembered the notes I'd made and gave them to her.

Chuck is now going into detail thanking guests for their kindness while Brenda was sick. The focus is on Donald, on Chuck's sister, on Brenda and Chuck's friends. He barely mentions me. Yet I feel I was there. While Brenda was in the hospital after the Whipple, I *was* there. I held a cool washcloth to her forehead when she vomited, spooned crushed ice into her mouth, shampooed her hair as she bent forward over the side of the bed, kept watch from the corner while she slept. She was appreciative, affectionate. Over and over, during her long stay in the hospital and recuperation at home, she said, "I can't imagine going through this without you, Judy."

Now they're erasing me.

Their third son, Scott, stands to speak. At one point, he reads from the notes "Aunt Judy" made the day after his parents met. "He's real good looking! And tall! And nice!" Scott uses just the right inflection to sound like Brenda. I feel everyone in the room twisting in their chairs to find me.

My steak and vegetables, salad and dessert, wine—even the night air when Henry and I leave Noble's and walk through the parking lot—taste sour.

We give Donald a ride back to Brenda and Chuck's street,

where he left his car. He praises Chuck's speech and Scott's, talks about how wonderful the evening was. He's happy to be an integral part of the family now. I understand that. But does he know what the evening was like for me? Did he even notice where Henry and I were seated? Bolts of anger shoot through me.

"How do you think *I* felt?" I say, turning all the way around to face him. I want him to see just how angry I am. My voice escalates with each word. "Did you ever stop to see, during this whole *won*derful evening, that Henry and I were seated in Siberia?"

"Judy, I didn't even notice." I watch his face fall. He says how sorry he is. That's the good thing about Donald. Nothing I could say would change the way he feels about me. Nothing he could say would change my feelings toward him. He cares if I'm upset. I care if he's upset. Evidence of what eight years' difference between siblings can do. Also, not being sisters helps. I reach over the seat to pat his knee in gratitude.

The rest of the ride, I look out my window at the watery ditch beside the road.

When we pull up beside his car, he gets out, opens my door, and hugs my neck. "I'm sorry, Judy," he says. "I'm really sorry."

"I'm sorry, too. You didn't deserve that. I got mad at the wrong person." Again.

On the way home, Henry turns to me and says, "I know how difficult this evening was for you." His words are soft, as though he's saying that great southern thing, *Bless your heart.* He puts his hand on top of mine.

When we walk into the house, there are messages on the machine from Laurie and from Mike. They're astonished at what they just witnessed.

44

In the early seventies, Brenda and Chuck and Henry and I attended Marriage Encounter, a self-help weekend held at a local college and promoted as an opportunity to "make a good marriage better." After the weekend, Brenda and I admitted to each other that, along with "encountering" our husbands, she and I had both found ourselves reflecting on our relationship. During the weekend, "lead couples" gave personal and revealing talks on different areas of marriage. At times, I saw Brenda turning all the way around in her chair to catch my eye. I found myself leaning forward for a glimpse of her face. After each talk, the participants returned to the dorm rooms where we were staying to "do our ten-and-ten"—ten minutes writing out our feelings on the topic, ten minutes reading aloud and discussing what we'd written. The goal of the weekend was improved communication.

Brenda and I could use some Sister Encounter now.

This complicated alliance of love and will, collusion and collision.

Scott, Brenda and Chuck's third son, is the family peace-maker. He calls to talk about his mother's and my conflict. With a neutrality that takes into consideration both his mother's side and mine, he tells me that his mother can't understand how I could make such a big deal over her reaction to my book, knowing it's been only two years since her surgery, knowing her prognosis even after surgery wasn't good.

I tell Scott that, in my mind, her illness and her reaction to my book are two separate things. In fact, it's hard for me to understand why she even brought her illness into this. I was devastated when she got sick and feel that I showed that by being right there with her throughout. My question still is, why was her reaction to my book so cold?

A couple of weeks before Brenda's December birthday, I decide to call and invite her to lunch.

She goes through her calendar. "Tuesday's out, I have plans. Can't do it Wednesday, we're going to the beach with friends for New Year's. The next week, I'm busy." Finally, she says she just can't make it.

I say I'd really like to take her to lunch and if she finds a free day, call.

Surprisingly, the week of her birthday, she calls and we go to lunch, on her actual birthday, at our usual restaurant. Our time together is easy. *We're* easy. Unencumbered. No mention of our recent troubles. We order our same fried chicken pieces over romaine salad, our same Roquefort dressing, not the vinaigrette

that comes with it. I give her a birthday present with an affectionate note. I grow hopeful.

But days after our lunch, she's back to frosty. If we didn't have
Mattie and her medical problems to handle (she fell, broke her
ankle, was in the hospital, now in a rehab nursing home), there
would be few words between my sister and me.

And then, frosty turns to angry.

We're talking on the phone one day, about Mattie, and I ask,
"How are *you* feeling?"

Her answer: "At the risk of using my illness, I won't answer
that question."

"What do you mean?" I say.

"You know very well what I mean."

And then my conversation with Scott comes back to me.
Why did I say *anything* to him? What was I thinking? Apparent-
ly, sometime between the birthday lunch and today, not knowing
his mom and I were close to reconciling, believing he could help,
he told her what I'd said. My words sounded to her like I was ac-
cusing her of exploiting her illness.

She's about to hang up on me. Quickly, I try to explain what I
said, what I meant. She isn't buying. Click.

I make another attempt, send an e-mail.

Her e-mail back, all caps, ends with: "I AM GOING TO
FORGET THE WHOLE THING—FROM THE BEGIN-
NING TO THE END—WHICH I SINCERELY HOPE
THIS IS. AND IT IS A SURE THING THAT I WILL
NEVER MENTION MY ILLNESS AGAIN—IN ANY
CONTEXT!"

We've crossed over into a whole new area, the two of us
trapped in something sticky, like a spider's threads.

45

When Brenda was sick, I would never have *not* been there. It's what I know how to do. Just by observing Mother all those years, I learned how to console, empathize, take care of someone.

But then I had a need. Not nearly as important as Brenda's. But not an altogether unreasonable need. *Because this matters to me, I'd like it to matter to you.* In our initial phone conversation about my book, my voice was probably glazed with insistence— because I was trying so hard not to sound insistent. After all, I was the baby of the family, held on that satin pillow, the one who grew accustomed to the kind of attention my mother was so good at giving.

I learned firsthand how to give attention and how to receive it. I did not learn what to do when I expected something that didn't come.

For Brenda, an expectation from me feels like coercion.

For Brenda, everything pales in comparison to dying.

For the two of us: something has been brought up from as deep as we will ever get.

We stay divided for a year and a half.

46

On August 28, 2005, she calls. Out of the blue. Her voice is relaxed, warm. Her heart has softened, I can tell. I don't lower myself to the chair. I don't loosen my grip on the phone even slightly. I hardly blink. I don't want to change the course of this conversation by moving even an inch.

She says she has just come from a funeral. A friend of Chuck's and hers died, one of three brothers. The remaining two brothers gave eulogies. She was extremely moved by what the brothers said. More than once, she uses the word *heartrending*. She describes not only the eulogies but the three brothers—this one's nature, that one's nature, each brother individual and distinct, yet linked. (Years from now, Scott will tell me that, after the funeral and before she decided to call me, she told him of her emotional reaction to the funeral and he asked her, as lightly as he could, no pressure, "Doesn't that make you want to work on your relationship with Aunt Judy?" She answered, "It does." And then she called me.)

The unspoken subject of the eulogies was the solid center that held the brothers together. The unspoken subject of our conversation is what's been lost and now remembered. I can almost see color rising in her face as she describes the purely ordinary splendor of the love those siblings had for each other.

47

"I've got really bad news, Aunt Judy," Brian says. It's Brenda's second son calling, September 14, 2005, seventeen days since Brenda's and my conciliatory phone conversation.

We've had seventeen days of normalcy. Conversations about gardening, about our children and grandchildren. Our annual shopping for pansies. Dinner out—Brenda and Chuck, Donald, Henry and me. Hugs when we greet each other. Open smiles.

Brian sounds breathless, although he's been robust and spirited since the day he spoke his first words. That adrenalized quality, usually so endearing, is scaring me today. "Mom and Dad were in the mountains and Mom started having excruciating stomach pains in the middle of the night and throwing up, and they drove straight back to Charlotte to the emergency room. They did a

CAT scan and found cancer in her liver and lymph nodes."

The air conditioning in the house suddenly feels cranked up. I open the back door, take the phone into the warmth of the screened porch. From next door comes the bass beat of a basketball against a backboard. I can feel the vibration of each shot.

My voice, when I answer, is the voice of someone about to cry. Liver involvement. Lymph nodes. This is illness on a whole new level. An image impossible to see around. For a second, I force myself to picture John, the boy next door, shooting the ball, his face flushed, those strong fingers spread over the ball, how he holds it so securely before offering it up.

After Brian and I hang up, Chuck calls. He tells me they're waiting to hear from the oncologist.

"What can I do to help?" I ask.

"Let's hold off till we see what tests he orders."

So I wait.

Did he say he'd call? Should I check back? Did he mean the doctor is coming by? Maybe Chuck is calling relatives and friends. I don't want to interrupt.

I wait.

My reconciliation with Brenda is so new, this situation so dire, the way forward—what I should do next—too unclear.

Finally, I decide I'll just do what feels natural. I leave for the hospital.

Slowly, I open the door to her room. Brenda's covers are pulled up to her chin. She isn't wearing her glasses, her face is pale and drained, and she's fast asleep. Chuck is in the recliner next to the bed, also asleep. Chuck's sister Doris, down from Toronto for the reunion they'd all attended in the mountains, is lying across two chairs, sound asleep. I quietly close the door, then scribble a note—my hands are shaking—and, because I don't want to risk opening that heavy door again and waking them, I fit the note inside the bracket that holds patient charts outside the room. In my note, I say that I'm sorry I missed seeing her and hope with all my heart the news will soon be more positive. And then I say she *is* my heart. I sign it, "I love you, Judy."

I drive down through the levels of the hospital parking garage—the rough music of cars overhead and below—making my way to the exit. The past fills my mind, the present, the future. Round and round I go. Now, then, tomorrow, next week. Brenda. Our deep connection. Her health. Is she in pain? How much pain is ahead for her? Can the doctors do anything? The two of us. Her *existence*. How long? Grief is clearly the subject. I don't want a sisterless future.

Something is hauling me back where we came from. The pictures we drew. The jewelry we made. Our neighborhood newspaper. The plays in the henhouse next door. The paper dolls and dresses and hats and blouses and skirts and evening gowns and tiaras we made and stored in cigar boxes on the mantel in our room.

Brenda and Judy. Like paper dolls. One so flimsy she might dissolve without the other.

Early the next morning, Chuck calls to say she is scheduled for an MRI. The doctor just left. Brenda would like to see me.

Immediately, I leave for the hospital.

When I walk into her room, I go right over and kiss her on the forehead. She's alone. I pull a chair close and touch her hand. Her hair is sticking out a little on one side, so I smooth it down. Though she's weighed down by nausea and dizziness and pain, she appears light, almost cheerful. She tells me all that has gone on, in detail. She talks and talks, as though nothing disagreeable has ever been part of our history. We could be children side by side in our twin beds, not ready for sleep, jabbering just before Mother and Daddy call in to us to turn out the light. We could be teenagers, shopping in the store, taking turns helping the other find something "cute." She could be a newlywed in Chapel Hill, and I'm hanging out with my *married* sister.

Chuck and Doris arrive. Then the transporter, a young guy with an impossibly bright smile, comes with a gurney to take Brenda down for the MRI. This is the test that will provide definitive information on the cancer. This is the type of marker you look back on: Before this test, life was one way. Afterward, our lives will be about whatever it is they find.

The transporter and a nurse help Brenda from the bed onto the gurney. He wheels the IV stand around, ready to take her down to fourth-floor radiation. The nurse tucks a blanket around Brenda's legs. Brenda signals to Chuck to hand her the pillow from the bed. Doris remains in her chair, back in the room, beside the window. Chuck is standing next to the gurney, now in the hall. I'm a little behind him, in the doorway, but I squeeze beside him so I can see her. She looks at me, reaches both arms up—as she and I have done countless times with one another throughout our lives. I bend over her, wrapping my arms around her and kissing her cheek. We both have tears in our eyes. This moment—even before we hear the results of the MRI—is a marker, too. The year and a half is definitely over. Our barriers are down. We're back to being sisters. Starting over from scratch.

48

The MRI confirms that Brenda's cancer has recurred. It's not that it has metastasized, as we'd originally thought; it has simply come back. Maybe that's a good sign—"recurrence" sounds less sinister than "metastasis." On the other hand, this just might be a characteristic of bile duct cancer, that it doesn't metastasize; it recurs. No one has asked the doctor these questions. Instead, we ponder the different terms the way patients and their families do, guessing what they might mean, wishing we knew more. There's been no further mention of lymph nodes.

Chuck takes Brenda to Johns Hopkins, where the doctors corroborate the results of the testing in Charlotte and present a plan. She's to have chemo (back home in Charlotte) every two weeks, a more potent combination than she had three and a half years ago with the Whipple surgery. Then, it just caused fatigue—not a simple, back-home-after-running-errands kind of fatigue, more a flat-on-your-back fatigue. Still, it was only fatigue. No nausea or hair loss. This new chemo will be worse: she'll be exhausted and nauseated, and her hair will probably fall out. After four rounds, she'll have a scan to see if the treatment contained the tumor (or even shrank it). If that's the case, she'll undergo radiation at Johns Hopkins, a very specific type that will pinpoint the remains of the tumor.

Thursday morning, October 6, at 8:45, she's scheduled to begin. I stop by the hardware store to buy her leather gardening gloves to show my belief (my hope) that she'll be back to a regular life soon. When we were growing up, being sick was an *occasion*. As if the whole world existed just for us. Mattie or Mother brought us meals on a pink wicker bed tray. Our family even had a separate set of dishes for illness—blue and white with a dewy rosebud painted in the center. The plates were smaller than regular dinner plates. "You just don't have an appetite when you're sick. There's nothing less appealing than a big plate of food!" Mother would say. I can still see her shaking down the thermometer, that whit-whit-whit. She always brought a get-well present—a book or toy when we were little, a lipstick when we were teenagers. Now that Brenda and I are grown, if one of us is sick, the other will say sympathetically, "Ohh, you need a lipstick." A few years ago when I had back trouble, she brought her homemade black bean soup and magazines. Two lipsticks, in other words.

The receptionist in the oncologist's office finds Brenda's name in the computer and points toward the double doors. It's an upbeat office. Halloween decorations everywhere. Large and small pumpkins, cats with arched backs, everything orange and black. No ghosts or skeletons or graveyards, of course.

Down the hall, past exam rooms.

At the end of the hall, the infusion room.

It's spacious and clean and white, lined with leatherlike reclin-
ers with extrawide upholstered arms. I wait for a boy with a wet
and serious cough to clear the doorway; he's wearing his baseball
cap backward and is pushing an IV stand.

Brenda is tucked in a chair in the corner. Chuck brought her
this morning and left to run errands. She's wearing dark slacks
and a white sweater set. Her left arm is out of her cardigan sleeve
and outstretched on the wide arm of the chair. I glance up at the
bag of cloudy liquid. One bead after another glides through the
tubing, splits open, and disappears into the hollow of her arm.

She looks tired, though I'd call it a tranquil tiredness. With
her free hand, she's eating a salami sandwich and potato chips. I
make a joke about the salami. It's not the sort of thing she would
normally eat. She laughs and says that lately she gets cravings,
and they're always for something with a sharp taste. The other
night, she says, she called her oldest son, David, who lives and
works in Charlotte (has been doing very well for years), and asked
him to make her his broccoli and soy sauce. It tasted just right.

"When they started the chemo, it was causing so much sting-
ing the nurse had to slow the drip," she says. "Now maybe it's *too*
slow."

I can almost feel the sting deep in my own arm.

The next day, Friday, Brenda and I talk on the phone. As she
was finishing chemo yesterday, she says, her blood sugar got out
of whack and she needed a shot of insulin. Which means the
bile duct cancer is affecting how her body handles glucose. The
elevated blood sugar made her dizzy. Not her usual dizzy, but a
different kind of dizzy.

I ask if she'd like me to bring her the chicken broth I have in
my freezer. I could boil some noodles to go in it.

No, she says, she still has a taste only for certain things.

"What can I make that you might want?"

"You know what I'd love? Your mustard-broiled chicken."

"How about if I bring dinner Sunday night? Chicken, butter beans, and a tomato tart? I'll get the beans and tomatoes at the farmers' market."

"Perfect."

The next day, Saturday, when I call to check on her, she tells me that all last night she was nauseated. She didn't want to give in and take an anti-nausea pill because each one costs over a hundred dollars, and she thought she should wait until she really needed it. But when she called the nurse this morning, she was told not to wait, to take a pill.

"Also, after I have an infusion, I'm supposed to drink three quarts of liquid each day for three days. Well, I forgot to start drinking this morning, so I tried to catch up by drinking a lot of water all at once. That made me even more nauseated. Now I'm eating saltines and sipping iced tea sweetened with Splenda." Her voice sounds so weak.

All day, I cannot stop thinking about her. I almost feel nauseated myself. I eat a turkey, avocado, tomato, and arugula sandwich and can still taste it an hour later. It's balled up in my stomach like a fist. Of course, the broiled chicken and fresh vegetable dinner I was going to take tomorrow night is off. Her stomach is too upset for that. What on earth can I do now that might possibly help? I'd been so happy—no, relieved—to have something tangible to do for her. Now I feel blank, useless.

I wait until around three to call again, and she says she's feeling a little better, that she's mostly in bed, dozing off and on, sometimes goes into the living room, where Chuck is watching football. Nothing else is on TV, she says.

After we hang up, I immediately drive out to her house

with my collection of Marilyn Monroe movies. Maybe *Gentlemen Prefer Blondes* will be a small distraction for her. When we were young, we'd sing and dance to "Diamonds Are a Girl's Best Friend." She was Jane Russell, I was Marilyn Monroe. She'd dip one shoulder, circle it, make her eyelids go heavy. I had Marilyn's whispery voice and mouth twitch down pat. We believed we *were* them.

Now I want to believe that if I concentrate, if I try hard, I can take away Brenda's nausea, I can drink the three quarts of liquid for her, I can keep her from losing weight and her hair and her life.

49

I'm talking on the phone with Brenda. She's had two rounds of chemo, two more to go. She tells me she's decided to take up knitting again. A red poncho for her seven-year-old granddaughter. Just two rectangles sewn together, she says. Easy.

"It's been a long time since I've knitted anything," she adds, "but yesterday I started and couldn't believe I remembered the basic stitch."

"Gosh," I answer, "that says something good about your brain. That you can remember after so many years."

"I tried to think how long it's been. And you know, the last thing I knitted was"—I know exactly where she's headed—"that sweater for you."

Brenda and Chuck had been married a year and a half. It was 1961. Chuck had just graduated from Carolina; Brenda had transferred from Georgia but dropped out when she became pregnant. Their son David was four months old. They were driving a back road on their way from Chapel Hill to Rock Hill for the weekend, when an approaching car turned left in front of them.

Chuck called from the emergency room in Concord, twenty-five miles north of Charlotte. Brenda's femur had been shattered and her two front teeth knocked out. David's leg was broken. Chuck was unhurt.

I had come home the night before, after my sophomore year at Georgia. My parents and I lit out for the hospital.

When I first saw Brenda, her face was bloody and she was essentially in shock from the broken leg, but she looked up at me, saw my new madras shirt and khaki pleated skirt from our father's store, and said groggily, "That's a real cute outfit, Judy."

David's leg was set with a splint, and he was able to come home to Rock Hill with us, where there were many hands to hold him—Chuck's, Mattie's, my parents', and mine. Brenda was transferred to a hospital in Charlotte, where she was casted from her chest down to her groin on one side and, on the side of the broken femur, to her toes. Chuck stayed in Rock Hill that summer. (He would start law school in Chapel Hill in the fall, drive to Rock Hill to see Brenda and David on the weekends.) I stayed home that summer, also. Mother rented a hospital bed and turned the living room into a bedroom for Brenda. The piano was her night table.

The two of us spent long, clockless days talking and giggling. We watched TV, listened to records. I made fake get-well cards from people she and I knew, and delivered them to her with the day's mail. From one of Mother's friends who was attentive (ever-present) when anybody was ill but totally absent during good times, I wrote, "Yours when trouble strikes, M. J." We played Scrabble, the board balanced on the edge of the mattress between us, Brenda turned toward me, my chair pulled close.

That fall, I returned to college a week before classes to prepare for rush. I was president of my sorority. We had skits to rehearse, props to build, lists of rushees to review. (This was when I still felt gung-ho, before I came to see the Greek system as silly and hurtful.) The University of Georgia did not allow coeds to wear pants in public, but since classes had not begun, my roommate and I thought it was okay to wear our Bermuda shorts. We went to the Holiday Inn for breakfast, and there at the next table was the dean of women, who immediately suspended us for two weeks. My father was furious with the school for having such a ridiculous rule. I was happy to have two extra weeks at home with Brenda. Her cast had been removed while I was gone; her leg had not healed; she'd needed surgery. She was starting her second period of recuperation.

That's when she knitted my sweater.

Brenda is saying, "I worked on your sweater for months!"

"I know," I say. "I still have it." It's traveled with me from Rock Hill to Athens to Atlanta to New York to Charlotte.

"You have it?" she says.

"I do."

When I hang up, I turn to Henry, who's been reading the morning paper across the kitchen table. "There's one of our problems," I say, pulling a limp sprig of lantana from the center of the table. "Brenda remembers how many months she spent knitting me a sweater. I remember how many months I sat at her bedside. I remember what I did for her; she remembers what she did for me."

I decide to find that sweater and take it to her. She'll love seeing it again. I'm curious to see it, too. Do I remember it correctly? Dark brown angora cardigan with mandarin collar. Oh, and the lining. Yes, I'm sure that she had the sweater lined in silk, so it was more like a light jacket.

To my surprise, though, I can't find it. It's not in my closet, hanging with the shirts and jackets, and not on the shelf with my

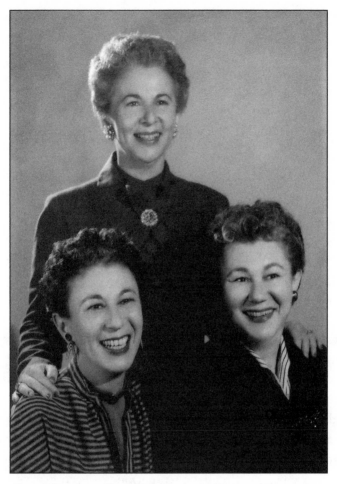

Our mother, Peggy Kurtz, with her sisters, Katie and Emma, 1955

sweaters. Not in the pine chest in the bedroom. Or the storage closet upstairs.

How could I have lost it? Did I give it away? Who in the world would I give it to? Where is that special sweater my sister spent all those months knitting, the hopes of three generations of sisters resting on its shoulders?

50

It's mid-November, a week before Thanksgiving 2005. Brenda just got home from the hospital. Three days ago, the right side of her body suddenly went slack, her leg started dragging, and she could hardly write her name. Chuck took her to the hospital immediately. After blood tests, brain scans, and an MRI, the doctors found evidence of three small strokes. I don't know if the strokes were a result of the cancer, or her treatment.

I drive over to Brenda's this morning to keep her company while Chuck goes to Costco. He needs to pick up some prescriptions for her, and as long as he's going, he'd like to be there around lunchtime, when all the free food samples are out. We laugh about this; Henry times his Costco visits the same way.

Brenda and Chuck's sons Scott and Danny and Danny's wife and son are all flying in from California next Tuesday. Brenda is planning to have Thanksgiving dinner at her house, even though she has pains in her stomach, her head spins, and her vision is blurred. She's also nauseated much of the time; her hair is falling out in chunks; she has no appetite and is rail thin. She's now on Coumadin (to thin her blood), and Chuck gives her daily insulin injections. A home-health-care nurse comes each morning to monitor her blood levels. Their son David will be at the Thanksgiving dinner, too, as will Donald, his daughter, Sasha, and her husband. David and Scott will drive over to pick up Mattie, who's still in the rehab nursing home in Rock Hill.

How Brenda is going to put on a Thanksgiving dinner, I don't know.

We're holding separate Thanksgivings this year. Henry and I will have Laurie, husband Bob, and their twins, Lucy and Zoe, and Mike, wife Brooke, and their daughter, Tess. It's the first time our "core" family has had Thanksgiving alone. We're usually with Brenda's family or Henry's sister's family. The reason Brenda and I will not be together this year is that we each made our plans this past summer when she and I were barely speaking, before a dinner combining our two families would have been possible.

As Chuck is leaving for Costco, he tells me that Brenda and I should have a bowl of barley soup for lunch. It's simmering on low.

But she's not hungry. All she feels like eating is a slice of raisin bread, home-baked by one of her friends. I have soup *and* raisin bread. The bread is delicious, and so is the soup—full of carrots, celery, delicate shreds of chicken.

I ask, "Who made this soup?" Her friends have been bringing food for weeks.

"I did," she says.

"You made it?" I say. "Wait a minute! Something's wrong here. Shouldn't I bring food to you? You're not supposed to be cooking for me!"

"But I love to cook," she says, "and I really like to eat what I cook. That's what I miss the most, just getting in the kitchen and fixing what I have a taste for."

"You like to eat what you cook. *I* like to eat what you cook!"

This is the kind of easy, jokey conversation we can have these days. Conversations that draw attention to the traits that make us indelibly ourselves, that distinguish one from the other, as well as the traits we share. For example, she says she "cannot eat without a napkin." Chuck teases her about wasting so many paper napkins during the day. I tell her that I don't like eating without a napkin either. And neither of us likes a glass too full, whereas our husbands fill to the rim. "When I was in the hospital," Brenda says, "every time I went to pick up the Styrofoam cup, I spilled water all over the bed because Chuck had filled it to the top!"

"I know," I answer. "If I pour Henry's orange juice in the morning, he jokes, 'Don't I merit a whole glass?'"

Also, we both always leave one bite of food uneaten on our plates. It's not something we do consciously; we just get full one bite before we're done. Also: Both of us like a certain type of bedroom slipper. Warm and fuzzy but with an open heel so it's not *too* warm and fuzzy—like the ones Brenda just got from L.L. Bean and recommends to me. "Here, try 'em on, Judy. You should order a pair. I bet they'll fit you." And sure enough, even though she wears a size eight and I'm a seven and a half, they fit. "See," she says, "they're a little small for me and a little big for you, but with bedroom slippers, it doesn't matter."

I hear Chuck's key in the lock. Brenda and I are still in the living room, where he left us two hours ago, her on one loveseat, me on the other. But now she's sleeping. Abruptly, after about an hour and a half of conversation, she gave out. I could see it in her face, how tired she'd become. And I knew she was hurting. She clicked on the Food Channel and we watched Sara Moulton.

"She's one of my favorites," Brenda said, pulling the mohair throw over her legs. "I also like Giada De Laurentiis."

And then she was asleep.

Now Chuck is bringing in the groceries. Brenda wakes up. He's bought the same deeply colored sweet potatoes from Louisiana they bought together last November. We'd kidded about them before he left.

"Get those great sweet potatoes from Louisiana," Brenda said.

"Honey, I doubt there'll be sweet potatoes from Louisiana this year," Chuck said. It's been only two months since Hurricane Katrina.

But here they are, smooth-skinned and smoky orange. Brenda tells me to please take more than half—she doesn't need this many for Thanksgiving, they'll just spoil. Then she goes into her bedroom for more sleep. Chuck leaves to check phone messages. I rip the mesh, spread the sweet potatoes over the kitchen counter. Fourteen in all. I count out eight, tuck them into the bag to take home, leave six on the counter for her. Is it my imagination, or is the overhead light flickering? Did I take too many? How many is too many? I put back one potato. That's better. Now they're divided evenly between us.

51

Thanksgiving 2005. Just my immediate family. Mike comes early to deep-fry the turkey in the backyard. When he lifts the bird from the kitchen sink to take it outside, we act as if it's as big as a humpback whale. Part of our Thanksgiving Day ritual is to go on and on about the size of this year's turkey. Someone will say, "That thing must weigh twenty-five pounds!" As if we never saw the actual weight on the wrapper. The conversation about the size leads to the conversation about how delicious this particular bird is going to be. I think our family has always stated the obvious. Of course, most families take comfort in knowing what comes next. *Oh yes, this is when I say such-and-such. And then you follow with such-and-such. We're on familiar ground here. No surprises. Smiles all around.*

When Brenda and I were young and Mother would drive us from Rock Hill over the Catawba River bridge to Charlotte for

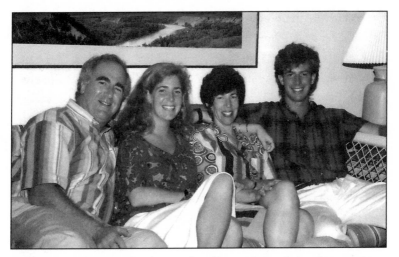

With Henry, Laurie, and Mike, Wrightsville Beach, North Carolina, 1991

a day of shopping, we would always comment on the water level. "River's high today," Mother would say.

"Really high," Brenda and I would echo.

Or, if the rocks were visible, one of us would say, "Boy, the water sure is low today."

When we returned home at dusk, we'd remark again on the river's rise or fall.

I sit cross-legged on the den rug and signal Brooke, Mike's wife, to place Tess, their nine-month-old daughter, in my lap. Brooke looks like Meg Ryan. Her hair is shoulder-length and highlighted, her skin smooth, shining, a lovely color. When she was shopping for her wedding gown, I told her to be sure to find one that showed off her shoulders.

Tess turns to me, full face. Her breath feels like a feather. Lucy and Zoe, Laurie and Bob's identical three-year-old twins, plop down across from us. Tess leans toward them. The twins (inventing a game on the spot, no conferring with each other necessary) bow their heads and pull Tess's hand to pat each of their heads. The twins then fall over backward. All three girls squeal with delight. Lucy and Zoe pull themselves up, hang their heads, and the game begins again: patting, falling backward, squealing.

"Okay. We're ready," Mike says, coming into the den, wiping his hands on a dishtowel. He's six-one, slim and fit. Not an ounce of fat. Strong. People are always amazed he can hit a golf ball as far as he can. He says he's finished carving the turkey. Brooke reaches for Tess. Bob, Laurie's husband, grabs my hand to make my push up off the floor easier. As I stand, I straighten one knee, then the other.

We arrange ourselves around the table. I sit upright and look at each person, how we fill the room. The tumble of our expanding family. I'm trying to remember something, where I am, maybe, how all these people ended up in this dining room:

Laurie and Bob met when they were at Duke, didn't start dating until after they'd graduated and Laurie was studying graphic design at Parsons School of Design in New York and Bob was back home working in Salisbury, Connecticut. They moved in together in Manhattan. Then they moved to Durham and got married. Laurie has her own business—Leap Design—in their house. Tacked to the wall above her desk are headlines clipped from Japanese newspapers. Stuck to her double window sill: a line of apple and banana labels. For my exuberant daughter, everything is brimmed with wonder. She loves chance creation. Bob programs and maintains websites, works for a company in Research Triangle Park. He has a smile like Lauren Hutton—that space between his front teeth—and he's intelligent, deliberate, and reserved. His sense of humor, though, is anything but reserved; it's all random association—and makes me laugh.

Someone has cracked a joke or maybe one of the children did something funny, and everyone around the table is laughing. When Brooke smiles that smile where she wrinkles her nose, I'm reminded of the first time Mike brought her home. They were juniors at the University of Richmond. It was the afternoon of New Year's Eve. She'd just driven in, and they disappeared into the den to exchange late holiday gifts. As soon as they were done, they brought everything into the kitchen, where I was cooking for company that night. Mike had given her a soft lilac sweater. She'd made him a puffy quilt—hand-sewn—and a collage with photographs of the two of them and love-struck quotes clipped from magazines. They perched on stools pulled to the counter, their faces shining up at me, Mike smiling his smile (which takes up his whole face), Brooke smiling hers.

We've all heaped turkey and dressing, rice and gravy, sweet potatoes, Brussels sprouts, and cranberry relish on our plates. "I have a toast!" I say.

Henry, Laurie and Bob, Mike and Brooke raise their wine-glasses. Lucy and Zoe raise their sippy cups. Tess is chirping, like a bird with a lot of questions, "Nah? Nah? Nah?"

"To all of us gathered around this table," I say, "my sweet husband, you young parents, these little girls . . ." I want to talk about generations, how things drift down through a family, how the world repeats itself—I'm just getting started—but I'm unable to finish because I choke up. I never get to say all I want because I *always* choke up. So, I just lift my glass.

Lucy and Zoe call out, "Cheers!"

More "Nah? Nah? Nah?" bird questions from Tess.

I mentally shuffle images and think of Brenda at her Thanksgiving. I hope she's having a good day today, hope she's well enough to be a part of things. I picture her dining-room table, once our parents', the light-colored wood with darkish whorls. I know the placemats she'll use, the iridescent olive-green and gold ones. Her table will be set with the china she and Chuck received as wedding gifts, white with black geometric trim. The center of the table will be given over to flowers I hope she was able to go out this morning to pick.

More mental shuffling. I'm back, Tess at my side. I'm remembering when Mike called to let us know Brooke had gone into labor, and Henry and I rushed to the same hospital in Charlotte where I'd given birth to both Mike and Laurie. We sat in the waiting area with Brooke's parents and Laurie, and we waited—and waited—each of us calling relatives and friends on our cell phones, saying, *No, not yet, still waiting*. And then, even when Mike came out, there was more waiting because he just stood there, star-eyed, unable to say a word. I believe his lips might have been moving slightly, but no sound escaped. In the pictures Laurie took, we're all leaning in to Mike, standing at such a slant it looks as if we could pull the words, one at a time, from his throat.

Finally, he spoke: "It's a girl! And she's fine! And Brooke's fine!" We were instantly damp-eyed and crazy with joy. Then he pointed two index fingers in the direction of the delivery room and again seemed unable to speak. He just kept pointing. Finally, through heavy breathing, he said, "I should probably get back."

The next thing was when we all crowded into the room where the nurses were tending to Brooke and the baby—plenty of nurses, very busy, and we were happily oblivious to the fact that we were getting in their way—and Mike held Tess and drew back the blanket so we could get a good look and we exclaimed over her awning of eyelashes and ripe-peach lips and took turns holding her and talking baby talk, the glassy music of that language, and then Brooke was telling how, the night before (eight days past her due date), she had made the special eggplant Parmesan recipe famous for bringing on a late baby and how, right after dinner, she'd gone into labor. Laurie or maybe Brooke's mother or maybe Mike was snapping pictures—I don't remember who, just remember not having to consciously smile because I was already smiling, couldn't stop—and Brooke took the baby, so close to her ribs, and we were even crazier with joy, that thick rush of something you can hardly think of a name for.

Concentrating on my family—instead of Brenda dying—feels like a pause for repairs, a suspension of time. The room itself is giving off light. I can think about grandchildren coming into the world, those honeyed moments, instead of my sister leaving. The arithmetic of family. The additions and subtractions. Like a Dr. Seuss book. People coming in, people going out. I can almost see the illustration on the page: Dalmatians wearing funny red and blue hats, walking on their hind legs, entering the house, exiting.

The morning Lucy and Zoe were to be born by C-section, Laurie lay in that high hospital bed, her clear smile, straight white teeth, thick and curly reddish-brown hair, which looks tousled even when it's not. Monitors were everywhere, sending out their secret signals. She appeared calm, those two babies curled just below her heart.

"It's time!" said the nurse.

Out in the hall then—with Mike and Brooke, Henry's sister

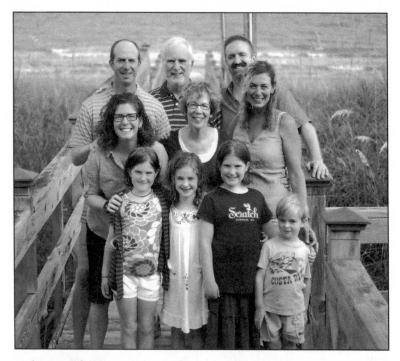

Back row: *Mike, Henry, Bob.* Middle row: *Laurie, me, Brooke.*
Front row: *Zoe, Tess, Lucy, Benjamin. Pawley's Island, South Carolina, 2011.*

Ruth, her son and daughter-in-law, Laurie and Bob's friends. Worries circled my head like drowsy flies. I left everyone to stand near the door, which we'd been told not to open. I joined the others again, then left to stand by the door. This time, I opened it a little. Enough to slip into the narrow hall, close to the double-swing doors leading to the OR of the labor and delivery suite. I looked around. No nurses to tell me to go back. Good. I stood there, glad to be alone, glad to give in to my fears and think of all the things that could be going wrong in there.

And that minute, through the double doors, I heard a baby's cry! Then another baby's cry!

When Bob brought out the two tiny bundles of blanket, we could see how truly identical the babies were. He managed to pull back both blankets with one gentle hand, slide off their knit caps, and we saw their coppery red hair. Electric, it was so bright. Beautiful. Exactly the shade Henry's used to be. Red, red, red.

"Wow!" we said, practically in unison.

"That hair!" somebody said.

"It's really something!"

"Holy cow!"

"Holy shit!"

Henry and I moved in with Laurie and Bob for the first three months, to help. In the beginning, we placed the two babies in one crib, thinking they'd just spent nine months squeezed together; they might sleep better if they were touching. I remember standing beside the crib, staring at those two sisters curled fetal, knuckling their small bodies into one another. I held on to that railing and wished they'd be close forever. Even though I knew better, even though I knew on some level that it's possible for sisters to be *too* close, I pictured them sharing bracelets, braiding one another's hair, playing piano duets, never being disappointed by the other.

52

Later Thanksgiving evening, after the dishwasher has been loaded, the pots left to soak, leftovers stored in the fridge, after Mike, Brooke, and Tess have left, David and Scott bring Mattie by. This morning, they brought her from Rock Hill to Brenda and Chuck's house for their dinner. Now she sits in the back seat of David's car, her leg outstretched, the ankle she broke in August resting on a pillow. Lucy and Zoe crawl around in the front, playing with the turn signal and making the windshield wipers go fast, then slow. When we ask them to perform ("Tell Mattie your full name!" "When is your birthday?"), they oblige but do not stop exploring the dash. We adults take turns joining Mattie in the back, as though she's Johnny Carson interviewing one guest after another. David and Scott stand beside the car, talking with whoever is waiting to see Mattie.

When it's my turn to slide in, I tell her she looks young and pretty in her red warmup suit. She has lost weight, so she appears much younger than her eighty-eight years. Her smile, as always, is elaborate, wide as the earth itself. "Oh, I'm on the downside of the hill," she says, "but that's all right, because you don't have to pedal so fast!"

She wants to know how my cornbread dressing (her recipe) turned out. "Not so good," I answer. "It tasted sort of sweet."

"Did you put sugar in your cornbread?" she asks. I did. "Well, that's what made the dressing sweet. You don't want to make that kind of cornbread." Of course! Why couldn't I figure that out? She's glad my sweet potato casserole (also her recipe) was good. I describe Mike's turkey, Laurie's gravy (her recipe), Brooke's cranberry relish.

"Tell me about your Thanksgiving at Brenda's," I say.

She says that she gave the blessing because she had things to tell everybody. "I told them we are all one. We don't know who will be here next year, but that's all right. We can't help that. This year, we're all here, and that's good."

The next morning, Brenda calls. She gets right to the point.

"You know those bedroom slippers I showed you?" She sounds rushed. On a mission. Something is bearing down. "The ones from L.L. Bean?"

"Yeah," I say. "I really liked them. I'm going to order a pair. Just haven't done it yet."

"Oh, good. I caught you in time." I can almost hear a grin breaking out on her face. "I ordered them for you. I wanted to give you a present."

53

This afternoon, Brenda has an appointment with the oncologist to hear the results of the scan that will indicate whether the two months of chemo contained (or even shrank) the tumor. It's December 1, 2005. I have an appointment at the same time for a haircut and color. It feels disrespectful—insensitive, really—to keep my appointment. But I would still need to pass the afternoon waiting to hear from her. It all feels so wrong.

The salon I go to is peaceful. The stylist purposely schedules only one client at a time, so that no one is waiting while he tends to me and I don't have to wait while he tends to someone else. The lighting is muted. There are chunky candles everywhere. He talks only if you talk. Usually when I'm here, the day stretches long before me like a cat. Today the best I can do is try to forget that this is the last hour and a half I won't know what's ahead for my sister.

As soon as I leave the salon, I pull out my cell phone to see if there's a message. Yes. Which means Henry tried me but the call didn't come through. I don't take the time to listen to his message. I dial home.

The news is not good, he says. Brenda has four new tumors in her liver and the tumor in her bile duct has grown. The chemotherapy was not effective at all. Hospice will begin this weekend.

Brenda and I knew. Yesterday, when I was at her house, she said she had a feeling the news would be bad. "If I were feeling better, I'd be optimistic. But the fact is, I'm getting worse every day." She gazed into my eyes without expression; nothing about her face changed. "That can mean only one thing. Don't you agree, Judy?"

So many times when she and I had speculated about her cancer, I tried to encourage her by reminding her of the "Uncle Irwin syndrome." Uncle Irwin had multiple health problems, all of them serious. He had half his stomach removed. He had total knee replacement before that type of surgery was commonplace. He had a heart attack and bypass surgery. Aunt Katie, Mother, and Daddy were all healthy. Meanwhile, Uncle Irwin outlived every one of them. "Maybe you'll be like Uncle Irwin," I would say to Brenda, "and bury us all."

This time, I had to answer yes. *I agree, Brenda. It can mean only one thing.*

It's staggering. Staggering how much I love her, how much she loves me. Staggering how charged the two of us can be with love, anger, hope. We're passionate about each other. Fixated. Anything but indifferent.

Well, what's staggering is that I'm going to lose her.

There is no measure in the universe for what it means to lose a sister.

54

My car directs itself to her house.

I don't ring the bell; I walk in. She's headed toward the door. The two of us, in one identical motion, synchronized and yet unintentional, lift our shoulders, hold up our hands, elbows to our sides, palms up. Our shrugs say, *Well, what can you do?* At least that's what I think they say. Maybe they say, *It's over, isn't it?*

The only words I can come up with: "My heart is broken."

For the first time in my life, I understand how a heart can crack in two like an egg hit against the edge of a frying pan.

I add, "I never use this expression, but boy, does this suck."

"Well, I'm sixty-six and I've had a good life," she says. "It's better to have a short life that's wonderful than a long life that's not so wonderful. Remember when I was first diagnosed? And Chuck and I made the decision to do everything we wanted to do? We probably spent more money than we should have, but we traveled to some great places and had a lot of fun."

She says she's tired—it comes over her quickly—and she

wants to go back to bed. I sit on the foot of her bed. Brian, her #2 son, is in the chair over to the right. Scott, #3 son, kneels beside the bed. Chuck is in and out; I have a feeling he's making phone calls.

The four of us talk. About the Thanksgiving when Mother was in the nursing home and Daddy was dying of cancer. How he was so sick but rallied because he was determined to put on that Thanksgiving. Brenda says, "He knew that would be the last time we'd all be together in the house."

Interesting that she uses the same words I use to describe that day.

Then she says, "He'd never been in a grocery store in his life, but he and Mattie shopped and shopped. Remember how he got so into it? That whole thing about the price of cranberry sauce?" And then her perfect imitation of Daddy's voice: "Too high. The A&P has always been too high."

We all laugh, loving our history.

She wants to sleep now, so I go into the living room and call Mattie to tell the news. I talk in generalities, no details; she doesn't ask questions. That shows me she understands exactly what I'm saying. Or rather, what I'm not saying.

When Brenda wakes from her nap, I describe my conversation with Mattie, how sad she sounded. Chuck is now in the room, along with Brian and Scott. Nobody speaks for a few seconds. Then Scott asks his mother and me, "How did y'all get through losing your parents? How do you stay strong? How do you keep from crying?"

"You don't stay strong," Brenda says. "You cry. And anyway, I'm glad you're crying. I would feel terrible if you didn't."

Later, Brian and Scott and I are in the kitchen. Brian is six-four, Scott six-six. All the Meltsner boys are tall and athletic. Everybody in their family is bigger than life. Chuck's mother had a sister, a large woman named Judy. Brenda and Chuck's boys called her Big Aunt Judy, the implication being that I was Little Aunt Judy. Standing here between Brian and Scott, I feel more like Tiny Aunt Judy.

Brian says, "You know, Mom could beat this thing."

Scott: "She's not going to beat it."

"You don't know that," Brian says. "She could go into remission. There could be a miracle. The doctor told her the chemo would cause her to lose all of her hair for sure, and she told me she didn't think it would, and it didn't. She just lost *some* of it. And nobody expected her to live this long after the Whipple surgery. She beat the odds before. Maybe she'll do it again. What about a liver transplant?"

"Brian," Scott says, "she's not going into remission, and there's not going to be a miracle or a liver transplant. This is it."

"Brian," I add, "the statistics are not in your mom's favor. True, she could live longer than the doctors expect, but when bile duct cancer recurs, it's not good."

I can see what's brewing. If I blinked, I could imagine Brenda and me having this conversation. The opposing viewpoints, the *lack of understanding* of the other's viewpoint. The way we kept catching each other being the worst we could be. I remember saying to Brenda, "Mrs. So-and-So is forgetful, and nobody is saying she has Alzheimer's." Brenda's voice still rings in my ears: "Judy."

Brian, Scott, and I talk, and talk. I tell them neither one is wrong. They're both just feeling thinned-out over their mother's impending death.

"Brian," I say, "you've been optimistic your whole life. All through school, you would think you made an A+ and were shocked when you got a B. It's your personality. And there's nothing wrong with that."

Brian is nodding and smiling. Scott still looks gloomy—well, maybe just solemn. Resigned.

"And Scott," I say, "you have some difficult decisions ahead, so it's important for you to look at the situation as realistically as you can. There's nothing wrong with that." Scott has decided he's going for his master's in counseling at a college in North Carolina. He could go to school in California; he'd be a resident there, whereas here he'll need to establish residency. But he wants to be closer to his parents and help them. His plan was to stay in California until spring, begin graduate school in the fall. Now he's not so sure his mother will last that long.

Scott is nodding. Brian is still nodding. They're nodding together.

"Your different reactions make sense, considering your different temperaments," I say, "*and* your different situations."

"Yeah," they answer.

"And let me tell you this," I say, touching their arms with my fingertips, "when your parents are dying, it's easy to expect your sibling to take away your pain and when he can't do it, you turn on him. Take it from me, you don't want to do that. Be patient. Be tolerant when your brother reacts in a different way from you. Do whatever you can to get along. It'll make it so much easier, I promise."

All three of us are talking out of our own needs.

55

Tonight we decide on the chicken and artichoke dish from Mama Ricotta's, one of Brenda's favorites. We always get the Caesar salad to go with it. Henry picks up the order on his way over. Brian leaves to have dinner at home with his family.

Brenda, Chuck, Scott, Henry, and I sit around the breakfast-room table. I'm keenly aware each time Brenda lifts her fork. I'm buoyed by the fact that she's eating. When the conversation grows lively, I see her getting tired. She pushes back from the table to go lie down on the loveseat.

Henry follows and helps her pull the throw over those long legs of hers. She kicks both feet out from under, just as our father used to do. Henry touches one bare foot and says, "I'm sorry, Brenda." She smiles up at him, cocks her head, and raises both shoulders in that shrug so typical of her.

Just before Henry and I leave for home, she asks me to exchange a sweater Chuck brought her. A white cotton cable-knit cardigan. It seemed like a great idea when he bought it, she says, but since she's no longer going out, it's a little bulky to wear around the house. She'd love to have something lightweight to wear under a warmup suit.

"I know you'll know what I want, Judy," she adds.

December 2, 2005. I feel an obsession gathering, like the way the air gets whirly before a storm. I'm gripped with the thought: why didn't I just end the conflict with Brenda—during that year and a half? My God, I had long enough to do *something*! Why did I waste all those months when we had so few left? Was I simply refusing to treat her like a sick person because I could not *accept* that she was a sick person? Did I want her to just be Brenda, my sister? Healthy enough to fight with. Healthy enough to hang around for a resolution.

Yes, Brenda was in remission, had been for a while. But we're talking about a form of pancreatic cancer. Everyone knows what that means. Why was I so concerned about her reaction to my book? Couldn't I just have overlooked it?

I didn't need to tell my side. I didn't need fairness. I needed my sister.

Her approaching death upset our alignment the same way our parents' approaching deaths did. Once again, the two of us were lost. Once again, I changed the rules and shrugged off my old, familiar role. I was not going to be the sweet one. Why, I could actually break with her! As for Brenda, the diagnosis of bile duct cancer showed us she's not invincible. She could no longer be her strong and brave self. We became unrecognizable to each other. Our *relationship* became unrecognizable.

Sweet. Strong. Broad words that never truly addressed the

specificity of us. What did those words really mean? The vulnerable one and the invulnerable one? The one with the self-doubt gene, the one without? The one who wanted intimacy, the one who wanted distance? Like Mother, I possessed the typically female ability (need) to keep the connection going. Brenda, like our father, possessed that typically male ability to hold another person at bay, to let a relationship drop.

Maybe the purpose of our separation was to demythologize our relationship. I know now we're no better off, no worse off, than Mother and her sisters, than Mother's mother and her sister. Than any sisters anywhere. The perfection of our relationship was just too much to keep up. All we are is real.

Maybe the purpose of the time I lost with Brenda was to prove to myself that I could live without her.

I wish I could say all this to her now. But I'm afraid it might boomerang. I'm not willing to take that chance. Somewhere along the way, though, I could have said I was sorry. I do that with Henry—simply find the part I'm responsible for and apologize, with the precise, pinpointed goal of resolving the conflict.

Now I'm left tending this small bundle of self-reproach.

Henry is working at his computer in his office. I open the door, sit down in the rocker across from his desk, tell him I feel driven to speak to Brenda about what went on between us.

I search his face. He opens his mouth, then closes it.

"I know what you're thinking," I say. "I don't mean I'm necessarily going to revisit everything. Maybe I'll say I'm sorry, that I never meant to hurt her. I just want to say *something*."

"Well," he says, "I would think it through first. Don't be in a hurry. Take your time. Get clear."

"You're probably right." More whirly thoughts. "I have something else on my mind—and this will make you think I'm really greedy. And materialistic. I keep wishing Brenda would give me something. Maybe a piece of jewelry that belonged to Mother before it belonged to her. Maybe some object from Mother and Daddy's house that is now in her house. I know how awful this sounds. My sister is dying and I'm like a buzzard, picking over her things."

"Wishing for that sounds pretty normal to me," he says. "It would be a tangible sign of her forgiveness. It would also be something for you to remember your sister by."

I think he's saying that I'm caught in the ambiguity of trying to let go of *and* keep something at the same time.

That night, Laurie calls to see how I'm doing. I tell her I may say something to Brenda about our relationship. I admit it's entirely selfish; I want resolution so that I can ward off any guilt I might feel later. I tell Laurie I might say how much I regret losing all that time with Brenda.

"I don't know that regret is what you're really feeling," Laurie says. "That word seems too limited. In fact, I don't think you should even spend time trying to come up with specific words. It'll sound too planned. But I also don't think you should just go in and blurt something out to her. You're really treading on thin ice here, bringing all that back up. Aunt Brenda doesn't like to rehash the past. You could just figure out what you're feeling. Then, if and when the opportunity arises, the words will come."

56

The next day, I go over to spend the afternoon with Brenda while Chuck runs errands. We hug hello, talk some. She says she's hungry, so I heat up the vegetarian chili her next-door neighbor brought over. I finish mine and take the bowl into the kitchen. When she's done, she places her bowl on a magazine on the coffee table and looks straight at me. "Judy, I want to talk to you about something."

I lean back against the sofa pillows and brace my feet against the edge of the coffee table.

"I want you to have my most cherished possession. And then, when you die, I'd like you to pass it on to Laurie."

She takes from her pocket the gold medallion our father won when he was a junior in college. He was eighteen at the time; he'd started college at fifteen. It's in the shape of an open book and has *Praestans Eloquentia—1927* printed across the pages. (After writing these words, I check an online Latin dictionary for the translation: "Distinguished Eloquence.") A laurel wreath encircles the book. On the back is engraved, *Awarded to Ben F. Kurtz—Junior Oration.*

I wonder if she was making the decision to give this to me at the exact moment I was telling Henry I wanted something of hers.

"I am so, so touched," I say, lightly fingering the scrolly surface. "I want you to know, Brenda, how much I love you, how much you mean to me." And then I take a huge risk. "We've had our ups and downs—"

"—but we're *so* tied in to each other." She finishes my sentence, shaking her head as though this fact still confounds her.

"Well," I say, "that's probably *why* we have our ups and downs. Because we're so tied in to each other. Probably too tied in. Things become intense for us, and we have to go away from each other for a while."

"I think you're right." She cracks one of her knuckles.

"I want you to know I never like being away from you. I did not mean to hurt you, and I know you didn't mean to hurt me."

"That's true," she says, resting her hands in her lap.

"I am very thankful I've had you for my sister. I admire you so much, and I've learned a lot from you. And I want to tell you something. In fact, this is the most truthful thing I can say right now: I cannot imagine life without you."

There was such an urgency to that last sentence, it almost felt involuntary.

After my conversations with Henry and Laurie, I didn't spend any time trying to figure out what I really felt. But something about having those talks enabled me to arrive at this simple and direct statement. And now Brenda has given me the opportunity to say it. Electrified is what I feel—because what I said was the most precise way to convey what it is to be me at this moment. She and I begin to cry simultaneously.

"Could *you* imagine life without *me?*" I ask.

"No," she says.

"See what I mean?" Now I'm teasing her.

"I'm sorry I'm doing this to you," she says, going along with the joke, which brings a smile to both our faces.

"Me. Too," I say, as though each of those words is triple-underlined.

The phone rings. It's a young woman in the neighborhood who wants to bring dinner tonight and also set up a schedule for neighbors to bring food each night. I check with Brenda, report back to the woman.

Now. Another subject I want to talk about: "What's it like for you, Brenda? I mean, what are you thinking, going through all this?"

Am I hoping she'll reveal to me the secret of life, that I'll be changed in some major way by what she's caught a glimpse of? Like that joke Donald tells about the man on a trek to discover the secret of life. He endures incredible adversity hiking to the village where, rumor has it, the guru resides. But then it turns out the guru lives on top of a steep mountain. So the man makes the climb, pulling himself up tree branch by tree branch, weed by weed. He reaches the top, is all cut up, has gone through test after test to get there.

"My son," the guru says, "how can I help you?"

"I've come to find out the secret of life," the man says.

The guru looks at him and says with great profundity, "Life . . . is a fountain."

"Life is a fountain?" the man asks, incredulous.

"Well," the guru says, "isn't it?"

"What's it like for me?" Brenda repeats, then laughs a laugh I can't quite read. "This makes me think of a conversation I had with

Daddy when he was so sick and living with me. I'd been taking that 'Alive' course at the Jewish Community Center. You remember, the one on interpersonal relations? Well, anyway, the teacher had been discussing death and how we need to encourage loved ones, who are dying, to talk about what's going on. There I was, armed with all that knowledge, and I came home one afternoon and asked Daddy, 'So how are you feeling about everything that's happening?' He smiled and said, 'That's the craziest question I've ever heard! How do you *think* I'm feeling about everything that's happening? I don't like it one goddamned bit, but there's nothing I can do about it, so I just accept it!'"

At this, Brenda shrugs both shoulders.

December 6, 2005. This morning, I start a letter I'll give to her on her birthday (December 26).

This afternoon, she and I talk about her birthday, about her turning sixty-seven. "Boy, we thought Mother and Daddy were so young when they died at seventy-one," she says. "Now I wish I could just *make* it that far."

Then she starts reminiscing about a birthday party Chuck gave for her years ago. We're not sure which birthday it was. Thirtieth? Thirty-fifth? Hard to believe neither of us can remember. We do remember Chuck filling the back of their old, broken-down van with their living-room sofa and as many chairs as would fit. He invited several couples and drove us from restaurant to restaurant—appetizers at one, entrées at another, dessert at a third. There was plenty of wine between (and during) courses, and everybody was red-faced and happy. All of a sudden, the yahoo of a siren—which sounded only like more celebration to us. But we were being stopped for speeding. The van could not go over forty, so there was no way the policemen—there were two—could ticket us. One policeman slid open the van's wide door, and out we all stumbled, unsteady, laughing and joking, balancing on the running board before stepping down, still holding on to our wineglasses. I remember the policemen scratching their heads. Somebody offered them wine: "Red or white, officer? We've got both." And then we snapped pictures, the two police posing and smiling for the camera, the rest of us pushing in around them like kids on spring break. We snapped pictures until we ran out of film.

57

December 8, 2005. After dinner, Henry and I drive to the mall. I want to buy Brenda's birthday present, Mattie's Christmas present, Hanukkah gifts for Laurie and Bob and Lucy and Zoe, Mike and Brooke and Tess. I don't know how much time I'll have as the days wind down to the end of the month.

What do you buy a sister who's dying? When I ask myself that question, I see her in the casket, which leads me to try to think of something that will last forever, something she can take with her, which I realize is slightly macabre. But I feel as though this birthday gift should be major, significant, historic even. Then I remember that Jews are buried in simple white shrouds, with no earthly possessions. Okay, the gift needs to be something she can use right now.

The last time I was at their house, Chuck was folding laundry and I saw that the gowns in the basket were the two I'd brought her not long before. I told her how glad I was that she was wearing them. She answered, "They're the *only* ones I wear."

I decide to buy her another gown. Henry follows me through the lingerie department, weaving through silk pajamas, woolly winter robes, racks of bras and panties. I look and look, but have a hard time deciding. Then I find *the* one. Lavender, satiny outside, soft inside, and warm. It has small gathers along the neckline, which are important because they will hide Brenda's mastectomy; I know that's a feature she looks for in nightgowns. I tell Henry that giving Brenda a lavender gown is just right because lavender was her first favorite color. I tell him about the picture she cut out of a magazine, when she was little, and pasted in her scrapbook. It was a room with lavender walls. She'd written beneath the picture: "This is the color I want my bedroom to be."

I look at Henry's face. Something is flickering in the corners of his mouth, and his eyes are wet. "This is the last birthday present you'll ever buy for her," he says softly.

We talk about the difference between this year's birthday and last. Last year, she was absent from my life. This year, she's present. But only for a short time.

On the way home from SouthPark Mall, I tell him that sometimes I picture Brenda joining Mother and Daddy.

"Do you believe in that?" I ask.

"Believe in what?" he says.

"That when we die we get to be with all the people we loved, who died before us?"

"No, not really."

"Well," I say, trying to imagine the millions and millions of people already dead and all the people just now dying and the logistics of matching loved one to loved one, "it *would* be hard to organize." I think about it a little more, and then my hospital personality kicks in—my belief that I can impose order on disorderly situations. "*I* could do it, though," I add.

58

December 14, 2005. Midafternoon, I walk with two neighborhood friends. I tell them that when I go to Brenda's, she wants to show me the notes and letters she's received. She is shocked at everyone's response to her illness. Actually, she's shocked at everyone's response to *her*.

"What do the notes and letters say?" one friend asks.

"They're very complimentary. They say how artistic she is, how smart, how she has achieved so much in business."

For example, there's the letter from our cousin Belle (Aunt Emma's daughter), which refers to that shy little girl who bravely walked into the beauty parlor in Rock Hill and sold the shell jewelry she'd made. That same shy girl, then grown up, who bravely walked into Lord & Taylor and Bonwit Teller in New York and sold the miniature canvases she'd painted.

I go on: "But the letters that seem to mean the most to Brenda are the ones that talk about how *sweet* she is. That's the exact word they use. And she's surprised and pleased that people see her this way."

"Especially since that trait is usually attributed to you," my other friend says. "And your mother."

It suddenly occurs to me that this is a mirror image of when I gave a copy of my novel to Brenda.

Yes, it turns out Brenda is sweet. Sweet in her own way.

Just as I am, in my own way, strong. I never thought of myself as strong, though. Even when I was twenty-one and broke my engagement three weeks before the wedding. Even during my first year teaching in Atlanta, which was the start of integration in the Georgia public schools, and my school (an all-white high school in a low-income neighborhood) was the first in the state ordered to admit blacks. Every day, there were bloody fights between students, police stationed on all three floors. I was only a couple of years older than some of the students, smaller than most. It was a volatile situation, but I wanted to be part of the changes that were taking place in the South. I didn't consider myself strong or independent two years later when I decided to move to New York, rented a room at the Barbizon Hotel for Women, worked my way up from production assistant at Filmex to secretary at Ogilvy & Mather Advertising to copywriter at Benton & Bowles. Then, after two years in New York, between jobs, I flew home to Rock Hill, met Henry on a blind date arranged by Brenda and Henry's sister; I returned weeks later for a second date; he drove his Volkswagen Beetle to New York for our third date, which was when we got engaged. Two months later, our wedding. Worked as a copywriter at a Charlotte ad agency. Then my own business. Two books of poetry, two novels.

But here's the important part: When my second novel was about to be published, whom did I want to recognize my strong, independent side? Brenda, of course. And now she wants me to

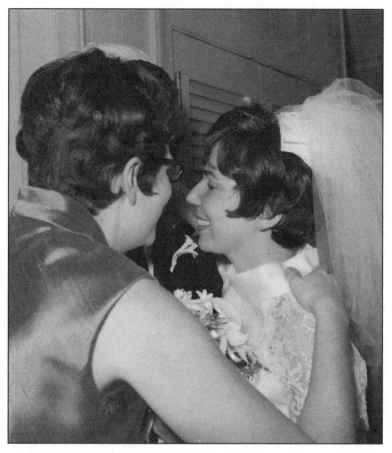

With Brenda, minutes after marrying Henry, 1967

see her sweet side. Deep down, she and I covet the other's signa-ture trait. Maybe it's time for the two of us to have the right to be both strong *and* sweet.

December 15, 2005. I call Brenda and she answers the phone. I love when this happens because it means she looks at caller ID and picks up. (She rarely talks on the phone these days. Chuck handles the calls.)

I ask how she's feeling. The methadone is controlling the pain, she says; Tylenol helps when there's a breakthrough. And while methadone makes her groggy, it does not make her as groggy as when she was taking OxyContin and Hydrocodone.

After this whole explanation, she says, "The saga continues."

For some reason, I don't hear her correctly. "Oh, I thought you said, 'The gaga continues.'"

She says back, "Well, that, too. The gaga *is* continuing!"

We laugh. Nothing of great consequence. Or even so terribly funny. But we laugh.

A little more talking, and we hang up.

I immediately start crying. I tell Henry, who's been reading the paper across from me at the kitchen table, that it's so odd how I'm fine and I'm fine and then, all of a sudden, I'm not fine. How some little incident will bring tears, as if a sharp and pointed thing has gone straight for a major organ.

He says, "I know exactly what made you cry."

"What was it?" I ask.

"It was that you had a laugh together."

That's it. We were in cahoots. Sharing a poignant, blissful intimacy. There's no one in the world I'd rather laugh with than Brenda. Because it zips me right back to our childhood.

The other night, at a party with friends I grew up with in Rock Hill, I told Ross, my high-school boyfriend, about Brenda's illness. His reply: "I'm so sorry, Judy. I really am. I remember how sad you were when she left for college." Then he added with a twinkle in his eye, the way people do when they've known you a long time, "You'd have thought she was dying *then!*"

December 25, 2005. I call Brenda and she picks up.

"How are you feeling?" I ask.

"I've felt better and I've felt worse," she says with a Yiddish accent, and a tone of voice that lets me know *she* knows she's saying something funny. "Like what Chuck's grandmother said when she came to the house on Eden Terrace and used the powder room." The powder room wasn't exactly a powder room. It was a tight and narrow L-shaped cubicle just big enough for a toilet wedged next to (almost under) a tiny sink, a washing machine, and a door that opened to rough and crooked stairs leading down to a basement that flooded every time it rained. Mother must have apologized to Chuck's grandmother for the bathroom. Chuck's grandmother's reply, in her broken English, which of course became family lore: "I've seen better and I've seen worse."

59

December 26, 2005. We all gather at Brenda and Chuck's tonight for Brenda's sixty-seventh birthday. The report earlier was that she was not having a good day. She was in a lot of pain, running a high fever, did not get out of bed at all.

When we arrive, everyone is on the verge of tears, and any exchange of words brings on those tears. Chuck has set the dining-room table with the olive-green and gold placemats, their good china, and little pots of African violets down the middle. It's so artistic Brenda could have had a hand in it, although of course she didn't. What is making us all feel smothered in misery is that it looks as if we're going to have a birthday celebration without our celebrant.

Henry and I have brought lamb chops, which he'll cook on Chuck's grill. I've roasted carrots and beets and made a broccoli and rice casserole. The casserole is not the best choice—it's sort of 1950-ish. Not exactly a green bean casserole with cream of mushroom soup and canned onion rings on top, but close. A few weeks ago, when I planned the evening with Brenda, every possibility I named as a side dish sounded like something she might not be able to eat.

Macaroni and cheese? I have a great recipe, I told her. Really different, not your average mac and cheese. Panko crumbs on top. Naah, she said. Too rich.

Potato gratin? Or even vegetable gratin?

Naah, too much.

I went home and searched my recipe file for a side dish light enough for her to digest. I came across this recipe for broccoli and rice that I'd clipped from *Cooking Light* and made when Brenda and Chuck came for dinner a long time ago. She'd really liked it then, had even asked for the recipe. (Younger sisters remember when older sisters ask for their recipes.)

We find our places at the table, with the chair at one end—Brenda's place—empty. Chuck, David, Brian, Scott, Donald, Henry, and me. Danny and his wife and son will arrive from California later.

The conversation is subdued. We all would go home in a minute if we could. No one wants to continue with this evening.

But then Chuck leaves the table.

He's gone for a few minutes.

He returns with Brenda, weak but smiling, on his arm. He helps her sit down—beside me—and even though her skin is greyish, she appears bright and ready to join in the festivities.

Something has lifted itself up that until this minute seemed beyond lifting. The climate in the room goes from chilly to balmy.

I am exhilarated, shiny and willing, the happiness I feel almost beyond bearing. As though I now understand about sisters. I could pull out audiovisual aids and explain to the world what it means to be close, how the ideal state of things for sisters is . . . not necessarily ideal. The ideal, in fact, is beyond the compass of most sisters. It was certainly beyond Brenda's and my reach. Our unreliable hearts kept us from getting it right. All our lives, we tried to make a dent in answering the big question about sisters, only to find that the final answer is: there is no final answer.

Everything is always more complicated than it seems.

What we shared is what caused us to fight: our closeness with our parents held my sister and me together—and pulled us apart.

Some people might say Brenda and I have made no progress at all, that we're still shadowing our parents. And maybe we *are* as stuck as ever in our same old pattern—Brenda facing her illness with strength, me showing that I care. I guess it feels like home to us.

Does it matter?

I have a hunch questions about sisters are as old as this circling earth.

When the serving platters are passed our way, Chuck asks me to spoon food onto Brenda's plate and cut her lamb for her. She says the meat is delicious and cooked just right. She loves lamb chops, she says. And she really likes the beets, they're her favorite vegetable. All in all, she eats maybe one baby carrot, a slice of beet, a forkful of broccoli casserole, and two or three tiny bites of meat.

I leave the table and bring back Donald's and my packages. "Do you want to open your presents now?" I ask. "Or wait?"

"Let's do it now!" I see a hint of play in her eyes.

I help her unwrap my gown, and she loves it.

Then she and I open Donald's bathrobe. She loves that, too.

She unfolds my birthday letter and starts reading silently. I realize, though, that it's difficult for her to focus, so I ask if she'd like me to read it aloud to her. Yes, she says. That would be great.

Under her watchful eye, I read directly *to* her, as though we're the only people in the room. It's a glorious, chiming moment. My letter is a series of vignettes from our childhood, which will later become an early chapter in this memoir: the two of us burying Donald's adolescent fantasies in the dirt; Brenda, flower girl at May Day; Brenda beating up the neighborhood bully; our playhouse, summer's hum.

Together, we slide into our faraway past, just as we used to lower ourselves into the swimming pool in our backyard, the water cool enough to soothe any fever. As I read, Brenda laughs, shakes her head—*Yes, I remember that*—finishes off some of the anecdotes with details only she can add. She and I started off together on Eden Terrace, and here we are—tonight—completing our journey, back on Eden Terrace.

60

December 27, 2005. I don't want to be away from Brenda's house for even an hour. I go in the morning and stay late. At the same time, I feel uncertain about being over there so much. I don't want Chuck to feel that his house is no longer his house. How much is too much?

December 30, 2005. Mattie was discharged from the rehab nursing home and is now back in her house. It's been a major struggle coordinating all the efforts to reinstate home health care, make sure she has her prescriptions and understands when to take them, get her the proper walker, make arrangements for her meals. For years now, Henry, as her power of attorney, has handled her finances, and I've been helping her with other decisions. When I was little, I made her a promise I would take care of her in her old age. I'm doing my best to keep that promise. Logistically, everything that can be done to make her comfortable has been done. Now my big worry is how she's dealing with the news about Brenda. I go over to Rock Hill to check on her.

We're in her living room, surrounded by framed photographs of her daughter, her three granddaughters, her great-grandchildren, photographs of my parents, my grandmother (Grandma Kurtz), Brenda and her family, Donald and his, my family. A stranger would not be able to tell whether this house belongs to a white person or a black person. And in fact, for as long as I can

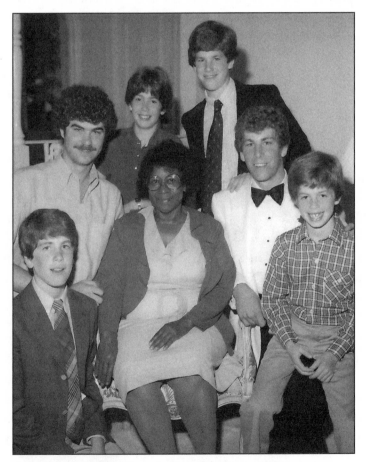

Seated: *Mattie Culp.* Clockwise from left: *Danny Meltsner, David Meltsner, Laurie Goldman, Scott Meltsner, Brian Meltsner, Mike Goldman. 1981*

remember, Mattie has introduced Brenda and me to her friends with, "These are my white children!"

Brenda and I have always gotten along well with Mattie's daughter, Minnie, who's four months older than Donald and lives in New York City. It's kind of amazing she's so open to our family. While Mattie was living with us, Minnie lived with relatives. She thought Mattie was just a caring aunt who came to visit every now and then. Mattie never told us this; Minnie did. Minnie and I were sitting next to each other at a dinner Brenda and I gave a few years ago for Mattie's birthday, and I'd asked Minnie about her childhood. There was no bitterness in her voice. Still, the idea that Mattie was cradling me, ironing my dresses, and combing my hair while someone else was doing all this for Minnie makes me feel worn at the edges.

Mattie is in her recliner, a slim pillow tucked under the ankle that was broken. All while Brenda and I were having our difficulties, Mattie never mentioned them. She didn't have to. Like Mother, Mattie believes sisters should be close. She has looked after both her sisters for years, even though her older sister, who now lives with Mattie, should be looking after her. I know she knows that Brenda and I are back together. I know she's relieved.

Now she's telling me that she lies in her bed at night thinking about Brenda. She describes a dream she had:

"Mr. Bennie came to me. He was wearing a light grey suit. I never saw him wear a light grey suit before. He always wore a navy-blue suit or a charcoal suit. Something dark. Not light. But he looked so good and sharp, and he was so happy to see me, and he was smiling that big smile like he always did when he saw me. I started to go toward him, but he said, 'Not yet, Mattie. Not yet.'"

"Do you think he was talking about you or Brenda?" I ask.

"I don't know," she says.

December 31, 2005. I walk into Brenda and Chuck's house this morning and call out, "Hellooo!" No answer. Quiet. Usually, Chuck calls back. I walk through the entrance hall, past the green and tan abstract painting over the narrow table, to the bedroom. First, I see Brenda, asleep, her face turned to the side and up, her mouth open. She could be eighty years old, her cheekbones are so pronounced and pasty. Then I see Chuck in a chair pulled to her side of the bed. He's hunched over her, his face hidden in the folds of her blanket. He looks stranded. With both hands, he's clinging to that lean arm of hers, and he's sobbing. The house is extraordinarily quiet and feels as large as a bank building, and empty and hollow. A husk. As though everyone has walked right out of here and gone on.

I pat his back, rub his shoulder. Without speaking, he points to three small glass bowls lined up neatly, expectantly, on the bedside table. One holds grits with a pat of butter not completely melted yet. One holds grapefruit sections he has carefully, artfully cut away from the rind, not one shred of pith. The third holds a handful of Total with a graceful sprinkling of sugar. Not a bite has been taken from any of the bowls. He lifts his face toward me; it's contorted with the effort of trying to stop crying. He shrugs hopelessly, as if to say, *Look at this. She won't eat a thing.* I know exactly what he's thinking. Up until this moment, he believed he could still coax Brenda to eat. If she were eating, she would keep living.

"See what you can do, okay?" he says. "See if you can get her to eat. And get her to talk. She hasn't talked all morning."

I touch Brenda's shoulder. It's as thin as a butter knife.

"Brenda," I say.

She opens her eyes wide and searches for where the voice is coming from. Finally, she focuses on my face and smiles. Her teeth are too big for her face now, like a badly drawn skeleton. "Hey, Judy," she says.

"Would you like some grapefruit?" I ask. "Chuck wants you to eat something."

"Pressure! Too much pressure!" she says slyly, joking.

"Well, how about pretending it's just very good room service? Like being at a Ritz-Carlton."

She smiles again. Chuck laughs. He's relieved not to be crying. I think he's also relieved the house is slightly less empty.

"Okay," she says meekly. "I'll have a little."

I tear each segment into pieces—flakes, really, each half the size of my smallest fingernail—and place them one at a time on her tongue. She ends up eating almost all the grapefruit in the bowl. Chuck watches from across the room. I don't know what this food is doing for Brenda, but I can see it is definitely nourishing Chuck.

61

January 1, 2006. Chuck calls at 7:50 A.M., saying he needs help. Brenda wet the bed during the night, and he's trying to clean her up, change the bed—everything feels impossible for just one person.

I rush over while Henry goes in the opposite direction to find a drugstore open so that he can buy Depends.

When I get to the house, Brenda is sitting on the chair beside the bed, naked, stooped over. She looks so bruisable. This is the first I've seen her mastectomy scar. I hate that my eye is drawn to it. I want it to go away. I want her breasts to be intact, like mine. She shouldn't have to go through all this humiliation with parts missing.

Chuck has already changed the bed. He asks me to wash the lower part of her body while he lifts her. She appears confused, definitely in pain. "I'm not really sure how to do this," he says.

I think: *it's the only thing he doesn't know how to do.* I've been constantly amazed at how adept he is at nursing, how gentle and good natured he is performing tasks that would make most men feel awkward, embarrassed, maybe even appalled.

Brenda and I have marveled many times at how lucky we were to get such great husbands. She and I are as much in love with marriage as our parents were. We can't say the same about Donald and his endless rotation of girlfriends. He always jokes that, when the first problem arises, he says to himself, *What do I need this shit for?*

I wash Brenda gingerly, shyly. After I soap her, how do I rinse her? Do I just let the water drip onto the bedroom carpet? I figure it out, finish the job. Chuck puts on her gown, gets her back in the bed, under the covers.

All night, she was agitated. She kept wanting something she could not articulate. He was afraid she would fall out of bed, or try to climb out, so he didn't sleep at all. This was his third night of not sleeping. Early this morning, he called hospice. The people there told him to give her a Valium-type medication from the comfort kit they'd left at their first visit. But it was hard to get her to swallow it. This is the calmest she's been since early last evening.

After he called hospice this morning, he called his youngest son, Danny, and his wife, who are staying close by with a high-school friend of Danny's. The friend's husband is a physician, and right after Chuck gets Brenda back in the bed, the husband-physician comes by. He checks her briefly, asks how she's feeling. She's able to answer, but is mostly quiet. As he leaves the room, he pulls me aside, looks me straight in the face with an intense and kind gaze, and says that Danny and his wife should not go back to California. They were planning to leave in a day or so. I know he's saying the end is soon.

62

Chuck calls hospice again and leaves a message, asking if they can come tomorrow, Monday. He doesn't want hospice to have to come out on Sunday, New Year's Day.

I all but pitch a fit. "We need them *now!*" I say. "I wish you'd told them to come *today!*"

"Well, we can wait till tomorrow," he says. "She's comfortable now."

Hospice calls back, and while he's on the phone, I position myself directly in front of him and kiddingly stamp my foot as though I'm having a tantrum. He and I both smile. He's been put on hold for a second, so I say, "Please! Tell them you've changed your mind, and could they possibly come today?"

He gives in. He's too tired to put up a fight.

Meanwhile, Danny, his wife, and their son arrive. Danny is Henry's and my godson. He works in the art museum at Stanford. He's European in appearance—longish sideburns, dark clothes. In fact, he once worked in a gallery in Prague, which is where he met his wife, born and raised there.

Within the hour, a hospice nurse rings the bell. The hospice doctor, a good friend of Henry's and mine, arrives right behind her. Henry invites him into the living room, where a football game is on TV. Danny and his son are watching, also. Chuck takes the nurse into Brenda's room. Danny's wife and I follow.

The nurse takes over, which is exactly what we need. Her manner is serene but authoritative. It feels as though she's bringing order to the center of our lives. First, she administers liquid morphine. She tucks the dropper inside Brenda's cheek, and Brenda swallows. No more methadone, she tells us. She says we should give Brenda morphine whenever she appears the least bit uncomfortable. She describes the signs of discomfort: A furrowing of the brow. Restlessness. A slight drawing of the mouth. She tells us that if we're undecided whether to give morphine or not, give it. The goal is to keep Brenda pain-free. We don't need to worry about giving her Coumadin. Morphine is what's important now. And we don't need to give her sips of water or food if she doesn't want them. We can swab her mouth with the tiny water-soaked sponges the nurse has brought, but—she smiles—this is more for our benefit than Brenda's. I imagine that if she had not come, each of us would have a different opinion on what we should be doing for Brenda. I'm so grateful for her presence. She then says that Brenda needs a catheter.

I'm afraid inserting it will hurt. "Does she need that for sure?" I ask.

"Yes," she says.

Danny's wife and Chuck leave the room. Just before I follow, I turn and ask the nurse if she'd like anyone to help, and if so, who. She points a finger at me and whispers, "I want you."

I like being that person. But I tell the nurse we should also bring Danny's wife back. She's been an important part of Brenda's care the past couple of days. I don't want her shut out now.

Danny's wife crawls up on the bed, holds one of Brenda's legs; I hold the other; the nurse does her work quietly and quickly and without causing Brenda distress.

The only problem is how to hang the catheter bag. It has to be low enough to allow gravity to do its work. Danny's wife leaves, returns with a wire coat hanger to slide under the mattress. Perfect solution.

While the nurse makes a phone call to start hospice nurses around the clock beginning tonight, I poke my head into the living room. It looks like a typical Sunday afternoon at the Meltsners', a group of tall males sitting around, watching the game. Brenda used to joke that on any given day, she could say "the game"—as if there were only one game in the world—and everyone in her family would know exactly *which* game she was talking about. Everyone but her.

I signal the doctor that he can come into the bedroom now.

He leans over Brenda, says with tenderness, "I heard you were rowdy last night."

She looks puzzled. "I was rattley last night?"

"No, rowdy!"

"Oh, rowdy!" She gets the joke.

After he examines her and asks her a couple of questions, he and the nurse leave the room. I hear the nurse ask him, "Don't you think she'd rest better in a hospital bed?"

His response: "Well, let's see what the next twenty-four hours bring. We might not get to that."

The nurse prepares to go. The idea that someone who miraculously turned this house into a refuge is leaving and we'll probably never see her again makes me want to run into the kitchen and bake her muffins or get her address so I can send a potted plant or, at the very least, give her a hug. Instead, I offer a skimpy thank-you and wave good-bye.

A conversation I had with Mike days ago comes back to me. About people leaving. About good-byes.

"Have I ever told you my theory about people, how we join together and break away?" he asked.

"Tell me," I said.

"Well, it's kind of New Age-y," he said by way of apology.

I laughed and settled in, loving this conversation with my son, who's a financial advisor and money manager, who's practical, purposeful, considered—unusually compassionate and sensitive and perceptive, yes, and open to possibility, but definitely not New Age-y. Past lives, future lives, tarot cards, and crystals are not what he normally thinks about.

"So here's how I see it," he was saying. "We each move through our lives. No, we actually float through our lives. Well, what we do is fall through our lives. As we fall, we hook up with another person, and another and another. Each of us has a whole cluster of people who are attached to us, falling along with us. Every now and then, someone cuts loose, continues falling but in a totally different direction. And because that person was attached for so long, there's a raw place where he or she once was joined to us. Some people who fall away leave an especially raw place."

"Interesting," I said.

"For example," he went on, "this morning, I was at the dry cleaner. Now I've been going to this same dry cleaner for about three years. The woman who works there is really nice, and we always talk. When Tess was born, I showed her my pictures, and now she always asks about Tess. We also talk about her grown son who lives in New York. Well, yesterday, she told me she's moving to New York to be near her son, and we talked about that. When I finally left, I turned around and said good-bye a second time. I felt really sad. She's someone I've had contact with once a week for years, and I'll probably never see her again."

At thirty-three, Mike is beginning to learn about loss.

63

Before the hospice doctor leaves, he, Chuck, and I slip into the small living room in the front of the house, and I ask, "So, what are you thinking?"

He knows exactly what I'm asking. "She's probably going to die within a few days. Looks like she's declining pretty fast now." He offers to return anytime we need him, gives Chuck his cellphone and home numbers.

After the doctor leaves, Scott calls from California. Chuck tells him not to come yet, there's no rush.

Before Scott went back to the West Coast after Thanksgiving, he asked me to let him know if things changed. This new state of affairs seems to fall under that category, although I'm nervous that I'm crossing a line with my interfering. Regardless, I take my cell phone outside and call. I tell him he should come as soon as possible.

I'm horrified to admit this, but I have a strong desire to take things from Brenda and Chuck's house. It's little things I want.

The flowery porcelain hand that holds a watch and rings taken off at bedtime, which sits on top of Brenda's jewelry box, the one Mother used all the years we were growing up. Who in the world would know or care if I slipped it into my purse?

Here's how I eventually give in to my impulse:

I'm in Brenda's office and see a recipe for "Mattie's Cornbread Dressing" on her desk. It's in Brenda's nice, fine hand on stationery from when she was an interior designer, maybe twenty years ago. As with all Brenda's careers, she started out dabbling and ended up with a full-blown business. Initially, she'd helped a few friends pick out curtains or sofas. Soon, she had an office at home with floor-to-ceiling shelves filled with catalogs and wallpaper samples and fabric swatches *and* client orders.

I want this recipe, this very recipe. On this thick, creamy stationery. I think of the cornbread dressing I made last Thanksgiving and how it didn't taste like Mattie's. Before I can stop myself, I see my hand tucking the paper into my purse.

Later, I'm relieved that this particular and peculiar manifestation of grief struck and vanished so quickly.

I confess to Chuck that I called Scott and told him to come. "I'm glad," Chuck says.

Chuck, David, Brian, Donald, Henry, and I gather around the breakfast-room table for dinner and talk about Brenda dying. David says he's unable to openly discuss what's going on. Donald says he finds it difficult even to think about it. Brian says his time is around four in the morning, when everyone else in the house is asleep. He says he wakes, starts thinking about his mom, and bawls.

After dinner, I'm alone in Brenda's room, sitting beside her. I like to be right here in case she wakes and is able to utter a few

Mattie's

Brenda Meltsner
Fabrics and wallcoverings
out of the ordinary.

Dressing

1 pan cornbread - crumbled.
1 onion, ~~chopp~~ grated
5 hamb. buns, crumbled.
1 t. pepper salt, if needed.
1 t. accent
1½ t. poultry seasoning
chopped celery

around 4-5 cups broth or
more -

Cornbread
2 eggs   350° - 425°
2 T. oil
1½ - 2 C. cornmeal
½ C. buttermilk
add reg. milk til loose.

Mattie's (and Brenda's) cornbread dressing recipe

words. Brian's wife has arrived at the house and walks into the room. I stand to give her a hug.

"You smell good," I say.

"It's Heaven," she says, raking her blond hair with her fingers.

"Heaven?"

"Yeah," she says. "That's the name of the perfume."

"Oh, I thought you were joking."

"No, that's what it's called. Heaven. From the Gap."

64

The next day, January 2, 2006, I call Chuck as soon as I wake up.

"I think the doctor was wrong," he says, his voice barely containing the glee. "She's not going to die in the next few days. She was awake and alert this morning and was able to talk for a pretty long time. She even ate some grapefruit."

The hospice nurse who's there this morning—a new one—told Chuck she's not so sure Brenda is ready to die.

"Well," I say, "the doctor said every person is different, and it's hard to predict."

Still, I am obsessed with when she's going to die. Originally, I just wanted to know how much time I had left with her. I didn't want to waste a single minute. I wanted an excuse to be at her house. A couple of weeks ago, when Henry and I drove to Durham to see Laurie and Bob and the twins, I found it wrenching to be two hours away. Now I want to know when she will die because I'm longing for her death, the same way I longed for Mother's. I don't want my sister to spend another hour like this.

January 3, 2006. The new, optimistic hospice nurse tells us that Brenda's body is shutting down. Her blood pressure is low. She's congested. Her breathing is labored. Her color is not good. She looks even less like herself. The skin on her face is thin and shiny, like the fabric of a skirt worn too many times.

By afternoon, she's unconscious. No one can rouse her.

Scott has been trying since early this morning to fly home from California. Twice, he's gotten on standby and come close, then didn't make it. Now, instead of wanting to hasten Brenda's death, I want to keep her alive until he can get here. When everyone is out of the room but the two of us, I whisper, "Hold on, Brenda. Everyone is here but Scott. He'll be home soon. Wait for him. He wants to see you again. Then you can go."

But every hour or so, the hospice nurse points to a new sign that she is fading.

I go back and forth between being fascinated by the ways the body declines to feeling panicked that Scott won't make it. Even though he was with her over Thanksgiving, I can imagine how desperate he must be to see her one more time.

Tonight, the rabbi comes to talk with us. He sits on one of the loveseats in the living room. I'm across from him in a chair I've pulled up. I dig in my purse for a Kleenex; this is going to be emotional. Chuck sits to the rabbi's right, in the recliner. Henry, David, Brian and his wife, Danny and his wife, Donald and Sasha (just arrived from New York) are scattered about on the other loveseat and chairs.

At first, everyone is hugely absorbed in what the rabbi is saying. There's a childlike alertness in each of us, as though he's going to unravel the mystery we've been witnessing these past weeks. But instead of revelations—or even alluring questions, about the shape and flow of life—he just talks. Actually, he lectures. About Jewish ritual. He could be teaching a Hebrew-school class or delivering a *Shabbat* sermon. I take a good look at him. He looks like a blind date; I opened my door plenty of times to guys like him. Portly body, chubby hands and fingers, mouth breather—allergic, for sure. I know I'm being judgmental, but I can't stop myself. Then I hear him say the reason he's talking so much is that he's hoping if *he* keeps talking, *we'll* eventually start talking. I think, *What an interesting perspective. I wonder if this new technique is catching on in psychological circles.*

But he does something that is inspired. He suggests we all go into Brenda's room and ring ourselves around the bed.

Chuck lies beside Brenda, holding her left hand. David stands next to the bed, holding her right hand. The rest of us complete the circle, holding hands. The rabbi offers a prayer, first in Hebrew, then in English. It's a prayer, he explains, to forgive Brenda for the times she may have hurt others.

I tell myself to listen carefully, take this in.

Here is Brenda's apology.

And here is mine back.

Is it crazy for me to take what is probably a routine end-of-life prayer and personalize it to this extent? At the same time that I'm analyzing, I'm also trying to listen to what the rabbi is saying. But I'm putting such pressure on this moment that I suddenly can't hear a thing. I hear his voice but not the words. I work hard, pick out bits of what he's saying, but then he starts praying again in Hebrew, and the words are lost to me forever.

Calm down, I tell myself. *Just find peace in this circle of people you love.*

Something inside me begins to rest. We recite the *Shema* together. Hurts, apologies—hers, mine—slide away.

I change my opinion of the rabbi.

When he leaves, I'm the one who walks him to the door. In the light from the porch, his face appears almost handsome. I even give him a quick hug.

65

January 4, 2006. Scott gets to Charlotte around two this morning. When I arrive at Brenda's house late morning, he's asleep. Chuck and his other sons, David, Brian, and Danny, are in with Brenda. I join them. The sheer floor-to-ceiling curtains have been drawn back. Even in this bright globe of daylight, the bedroom is pastel. Through the windows overlooking the backyard, I can see Brenda's hydrangeas. Over the years, she planted dozens of varieties. The branches are bare, wiry now that it's winter. They're not even close to being ready to put out new leaves. If you didn't know anything about hydrangeas, you'd think they were half gone. But to gardeners, this emptiness—the sculpture of the branches—is as beautiful as the summer flowers. And of course, the twigs bring birds.

Around noon, David and Brian leave for work, and Chuck, Danny, Mike, and I eat chicken sandwiches in the kitchen. For weeks now, Mike has been doing everything he can to shore me up, including leaving his office today to be here. I sit right beside him at the table, my chair leg in line with his chair leg. At times, we all talk. At times, the only thing you hear is somebody twirling the ice in a glass.

All afternoon, different ones of us go into Brenda's room. To-day, for the first time, I'm finding it hard to stay in there. I just want it to be over. *When? Hurry up. It's enough. I don't want this for you. Go.*

I pester the hospice nurse with questions, all skirting the one I'm afraid to ask: *When will she die?* I imagine the nurse writing in those pages of notes, which I can't quite worm my way close enough to read: Sister is strange and seems to want patient to die. I'm tired of her endless queries.

And in fact, the next nurse to come, the night nurse, teases me about my questions and is now calling me Brenda's "fussy sis-ter"—as in, "Okay, Brenda, here comes your fussy sister!" I laugh it off, thinking if Brenda were conscious, she might say, *You're right about that. She's my fussy sister.*

After dinner, Chuck and I clean up the kitchen. I rinse the plates and glasses. He fits them into the dishwasher. We hardly talk. We don't look the other's way. Neither of us wants to see what the other's face is doing.

Around nine, I lift the sheet and feel Brenda's feet. They've been warm up until now, but they suddenly feel cool, as though they're partway in the grave. I tell the nurse. She feels them and looks at the soles of Brenda's feet, then studies her face and chest. She rushes from the room and returns with Chuck. By this time, everyone is here and crowding into the bedroom—Henry, David, Brian and his wife, Scott, Danny and his wife, Donald and Sasha, Chuck's sister Doris, who flew in this afternoon from Toronto. The nurse tells us the end is near; she has obviously told Chuck this. He says he'd like a few moments alone with Brenda. He closes the door, and all of us cluster outside in the entrance hall. I sit on the stairs. No one speaks. Chuck is in there a long time.

Finally, he opens the door and waves us in. The boys move close to Brenda. The rest of us stay off to the side. We wait. And watch. There are spaces between her breaths, but the next breath keeps coming. The breaths are distinct. They sound almost deliberate, like the ones you take when the doctor, listening to your chest with a stethoscope, tells you to breathe deeply and then do it again. That's the rhythm of her breaths. Quick. Sharp. But rooted down deep in her body.

Scott asks if we could form a circle again, since he missed last night's. He lies on the bed next to his mother and holds her left hand. Chuck stands beside the bed and holds her right hand. Instead of a rabbi's prayers, tonight each of us speaks directly to Brenda, not in any order, randomly, some of us more than once.

"I love you, Brenda," I say. And then I say it again.

Henry says, "Brenda, I'll always be grateful to you because you're the one who introduced me to Judy."

Donald says how glad he is that he made the move from New York to Charlotte. "It means I've been able to hang out with you guys all these years."

Each person's comments are personal and loving. Most of us are crying.

This will be the last time we'll all be together like this. With Brenda.

Afterward, we drop hands but stay where we are in the circle and wait and watch. Her determined heart does not stop beating.

Finally, around eleven, Danny and his wife and son leave for their friends' house. Brian and his wife leave for home. Chuck and Scott are in the living room. The hospice nurse is somewhere in the house, not in the bedroom. Henry and I are alone with Brenda. Henry is sitting in a chair in the corner, and I'm in the chair close to the bed. I take her hand. Her fingernails are shaped and polished, a pale pink. I remember, maybe a week ago, one of her friends gave her a manicure.

"Brenda, everyone is here." My voice is low and straightforward. "Your boys are going to be fine. You don't need to worry about them. They're great kids. And Chuck is going to be fine, too."

I pause, glance up at Henry. He nods yes, keep going.

"I'll miss you, Brenda. More than I could ever say. But you can go whenever it's time." And then, rephrasing lines from "Caroline," a poem by Linda Pastan, I add, "When it grows cold enough, just button your coat and go."

The nurse returns to the room. I'm crying again. Henry and I tell Chuck good night and each give him a hug. He takes a sleeping pill and heads upstairs to bed.

Henry and I go home.

At 12:30, the phone rings. I'm lying in bed, reading, trying to get sleepy. Henry is at his computer upstairs. We both pick up. We know it'll be Chuck's deep voice.

"She's gone," he says.

It turns out Scott was with Brenda at the moment of death.

Scott, wanting to be alone for a few minutes, had left her room and was in the living room watching TV. The nurse came for him: "Hurry, she's going."

He asked the nurse to please call upstairs to his father. Meanwhile, Scott climbed into bed beside Brenda, rested on his knees, held her. All of a sudden, she appeared to be gasping for air, choking. She opened her eyes very wide, in astonishment, although it was obvious she couldn't see him. And then she just did not take the next breath.

66

January 5, 2006. I call Chuck this morning, and he tells me we're meeting with the rabbi at one o'clock. Everything having to do with Brenda's funeral is being handled by the rabbi and members of the Jewish community, as though some sort of external motion has already begun. I can almost hear cylinders cranking, gears grinding, pulleys hoisting. An apparatus is in place, specific tasks taken care of, one by one. Reserving the temple, contacting the cantor, ordering flowers for the altar, arranging for volunteers from the synagogue to wash and dress and sit with the body from the time of death until the funeral, planning lunch at Chuck's afterward, arranging for shivah (the formal mourning period). There've been times I've questioned the idea of organized religion. But I have to say, at this point, I appreciate the organized part.

And now we're sitting around Brenda and Chuck's breakfast-room table—the same rabbi who came two nights ago, Chuck, his sons and their wives, Donald and me—finalizing plans for the service. Henry and Chuck's sister are at the cemetery checking on the grave site. Scott says that he or one of his brothers will try to speak. Chuck says he will speak.

The rabbi says, "Chuck, I'll tell you what I say to everyone who wants to speak at a spouse's funeral: it's not like anything else you've ever done. I even tell lawyers it's not like speaking in court."

Scott refers to how tearful Chuck became earlier when he told the rabbi that Brenda could take plain chicken and turn it into a gourmet meal: "Dad, you can't even talk about chicken breasts without crying. How are you going to do this?"

Chuck says, "I can do it."

I say, "Scott, your dad can do it."

"Aunt Judy, you're going to speak, right?" one of the boys says.

I ask the rabbi if I can have the option of waiting until just before the service to make my decision. His warning got to me.

The rabbi says that will be fine. Then he adds, "Or . . . you could just hand me your speech and I'll deliver it."

"No," I say, a little more forcefully than I intend. "I know I won't do that. If I don't deliver it, I don't really want anyone else to."

"Okay, okay," he says, lifting his palms as if to ward off whatever energy I might be thrusting his way.

Our brief romance is over. I think I probably sounded rude.

67

January 6, 2006. The day of the funeral. I haven't slept in too many nights to count. I've got a cold. My voice is just about gone. I feel hazy. Tired. Need propping up. I have to take the day slowly.

Laurie, Bob, Lucy, and Zoe are staying with us. Laurie leaves early to observe at a preschool for the girls for next fall. They're moving from Durham to Charlotte this summer. Bob is trying hard to take care of the girls and relieve me of any responsibility. He's being quietly helpful. I open the refrigerator to take out orange juice and he sweeps in behind me, scoops up the carton, and fills their sippy cups. I ask Henry if it's too early for me to start getting dressed for the funeral. He says no, it's not too early. I'm the one who's always on time, and he's the one who's always late. He thinks that if we're invited to someone's house at eight, it means he should start getting ready at eight. But this morning, he's the one I'll depend on to tell me how to budget time.

I put on a purple-ish turtleneck sweater and black pantsuit. It's what I'd planned to wear. But when I look in the mirror, I see that, between the last time I wore the suit and this morning, it went out of style. The shoulder pads are too big and the jacket too long. The turtleneck makes my double chin triple. Hoping I'm wrong and my outfit is really just fine, I walk into the kitchen and ask Henry what he thinks. He shakes his head, says it doesn't look so great. Now what? I have no idea what to wear to my sister's funeral. If it were my funeral, she would have just the right outfit.

I pull out my lavender suede jacket, my lavender silk sweater, and my taupe pants. Around my neck, I hang my father's medallion, the one Brenda gave me. (Later, when I look around the synagogue during the service, it will be obvious I'm the only woman in the entire place not wearing black and one of the few wearing pants.)

Everyone is ready. Suits, ties, good shoes. Heavy coats. We leave Lucy and Zoe with my two neighborhood friends. Zoe is crying hysterically. I'm worried about her but don't want to let my dismay take over. I could easily let anything take over.

Mattie made the decision not to come. She said she wouldn't be able to take Brenda's funeral. I'll miss her, but I feel that she's doing the right thing. Mike and Brooke pick up Laurie and Bob, and the four of them follow Henry and me to Temple Israel.

When we walk in, the first people I see are Betsy and Hugh Rock and Kathryne Perrill, my oldest friends. We started together in nursery school in Rock Hill and have been close ever since. Seeing them, I feel my entire childhood taking shape right here in the vestibule of the synagogue. They envelop me in their arms and talk about Brenda and are sympathetic and consoling. I tell them not to say anything nice. I feel that if I can keep from crying before the service, I might be able to make it through my talk.

Then I see my cousin Debbie. My friend Judy Pera. Someone who grew up on Myrtle Drive, one street over from Eden Terrace. With each new person, I have to stiffen again, hold back the tears.

How in the world am I going to get through this? I never should have agreed to speak. I keep reminding myself I can back out at any point.

The family gathers in the chapel. The rabbi pins a black ribbon on each of our jackets. Then he instructs us to tear them—a sign, he says, that someone has been torn from our midst. I remember finding in the drawer of Mother's bedside table the torn ribbon she had worn at her father's funeral. It killed me that my mother could be so bereft she'd save the ribbon. I never could bear my mother's sadness. I decide then and there to throw this ribbon away after the funeral. I don't want my children to find it years from now.

We're led into the sanctuary. It's filled with people. Even up in the balcony. Brenda would be touched. I see Ross, my high-school boyfriend, and his wife. There's a row of Brenda's high-school friends. My main preoccupation, though, is to keep my emotions at bay. I concentrate on the stained-glass windows. The temple is new, so the windows are new. I hate them. Why can't synagogues have old stained-glass windows? Churchly ones. Why do we have to have modern everything? Why can't we have mahogany pews? I want Colonial or Georgian. Not contemporary. It's working. I don't look at the casket in front of me, slightly to the right. I just keep hating those stained-glass windows.

Suddenly, I realize the service has begun. The rabbi is chanting in Hebrew. Then he makes a few opening remarks, explaining the order of the service, including an introduction of the speakers: Brenda's sister, her sons, her husband.

He nods at me.

68

I rise from my seat, walk slowly and carefully up the steps to the altar, take my place behind the huge wooden podium, unfold the pages of my speech.

I cannot say a word. Tears are forming. If I open my mouth, I'll start crying.

I look up. It's quiet. And bright. All that sunlight pouring through the windows. Now I see that this stained glass has its own beauty and righteousness.

And then, in the wake of all that has gone on since Brenda's cancer recurred, I start speaking:

> Brenda, I think I must have begun to adore you the min-
> ute Mother and Daddy brought me home from the hospital
> and I saw you for the first time. Then we were beginning a life
> together. Now we're looking at ending a life together. Tender
> memories are swimming up, as if in shallow water.
>
> You're the one who sat for hours at the card table in the

den on Eden Terrace, placing tiny seashells in intricate flower patterns, turning them into earrings and pins. That was me sitting next to you, copying your every move, marveling at your artistic talent and business sense—qualities nameless to us then but irrevocably yours.

You're the one who built a fishpond in our backyard. You were so young—yet you poured the concrete yourself. Our parents might have wondered about that big, gluey hole in the middle of the yard, but now we know you were just demonstrating an early aptitude for landscaping.

You're the one who cooked with Mattie in the kitchen. Your peanut butter fudge. Your candy apples, which were so hard we had to crack them over the backs of wooden chairs to get them started.

You and I were always together. When Donald was supposed to baby-sit for us but forgot and asked his girlfriend out on a date, Daddy insisted he take us along. There we were at the drive-in, Donald and Mary Moore Sanders in the back seat, you and me in the front. All evening, we were adjusting the rearview mirror—and believe me, we saw a better movie in that mirror than anyone saw on the screen.

You were so much like our father—smart, wonderfully strong and steadfast and certain, **head**strong, brave (fearless, really), artistic, able to set a goal and achieve it. And you looked like him—that naturally curly hair, those green eyes, long legs. Like him, you were very sick before Thanksgiving, but you mustered every bit of strength you had to put on a magnificent Thanksgiving because you—like Daddy—knew it would be the last time your family would all be together in that house. Like **his** illness, **your** illness took a dramatic turn for the worse New Year's Eve. And like him, you breathed your last breath four days later.

But even though everyone thought you were so like him, you were also like Mother—that extraordinary sense of style, *not only in your clothes, but in the homes you created. Your sculpted flower arrangements, the gardens you designed and tended. Like Mother, you were pretty, graceful. Sweet.*

Brenda, you were the one I shared a room with until the day you left for college. You and I were talking about that room as recently as eleven days ago—trying to recall every drawer. Of course, you had your dresser and I had mine. The one drawer we shared held our neckerchiefs and angora collars, the only clothes we could both wear, and of course those were the ones we fought over. But we loved our room—the bachelor-button wallpaper, the working fireplace, the tall brass lamp that separated our beds.

A few weeks ago, I had been walking with neighborhood friends and we'd parted halfway. I was heading back home alone. The days were growing shorter, so it was already turning dark. I looked up at the sky. The moon hung just over the houses, and there was a hazy ring around it, which meant we'd probably have rain the next day. All of a sudden, without any forethought or self-consciousness, I heard myself say out loud, as though I had this amazing and joyful news which I'd almost forgotten to tell: "Mother and Daddy, Brenda's coming!"

Next: David, Brian, Scott, and Danny walk up to the podium, and Scott steps to the microphone to read. I'm proud of the four of them. Brenda would be, too. In their dark suits and ties, they appear poised, confident. Early in his talk, Scott tells an old family story about his mom punishing him and Danny, probably for fighting. While the two of them were banished to their shared bedroom, one asked the other, "Do you like Mom?" The other answered, "Naah."

At the end of his talk, Scott—with an affectionate nod toward his mom, whose presence I feel—refers back to that story: "And now I ask my brothers, do you like Mom?"

Then Chuck speaks. He wants to tell us a love story, he says. His speech is emotional and packed and detailed. He *is* able to say all that he wants to say without breaking down. His pain, though, seems prismatic, like the rays of the sun shooting through those windows. How appropriate for them to be refracted through cracked glass.

The rest of the service I cannot remember. The rabbi speaks, the cantor chants, we read in unison, we stand, we sit. I look at the casket and try as hard as I can to picture Brenda lying inside.

Then it's over, and the family is ushered out of the temple as the rabbi follows behind, reading the Twenty-third Psalm. The psalm is a wave we ride, surfing those words up the aisle. The psalm carries us out of the sanctuary, through the vestibule, all the way out to the parking lot and our cars. It's a bitter-cold day. This is the first I've realized I left my coat on the kitchen table.

Henry, Donald, and I drive together to the cemetery. We talk about Brenda. We're lost in remembering.

69

When I get out of the car at the cemetery, Laurie says, "Here, Mom," and helps me into her black coat. She slips into Bob's. We take our places under the canopy. I bend my body against the wind, hunch my shoulders so that the collar comes up around my face, and I stare at the hole. The rabbi drops a tablespoon of soil from Jerusalem into each of our palms, and we take turns stepping forward and sprinkling it over the casket.

The rabbi prays and chants. Every word echoes.

Then he offers each of us the shovel and says that the first scoops of earth should be delivered with the back of the shovel because we're not building anything.

Chuck and his sons go first. When Donald takes the shovel, I smile in spite of myself because he's never held a shovel in his life and, by mistake, he scatters dirt all over the bands crisscrossing the hole. Now he's trying to correct his mistake by knocking the dirt off the bands, but it's not working.

Henry whispers to me, "Do you want to take a turn shoveling dirt?" I shake my head no. He asks if I want him to do it for me.

I shake my head no again. I don't want to shovel dirt on Brenda's casket. I'm not ready for that part. There are other family members stepping forward.

The sound of the dirt dropping on the casket, over and over—it could be falling from a great distance.

After the service, several friends stop me to talk. My hands are balled up in my coat pockets. Nearby, I hear Laurie and Mike planning a bowling outing with their cousins tonight. That feels right. I head for the car. Henry has left the doors unlocked—he and Donald are still visiting with people—and I slide in the front. I'm alone in the car, watching the grave site. The cemetery workers are shoveling in the rest of the dirt, filling the hole. They work fast. Their shoveling is definitely not symbolic. They mean business.

This place is cold and lonely and far from Brenda's neighborhood and mine. Once again, I hear myself speak out loud when there's no logical reason to be speaking out loud. As though a voice were coming from the dash or roof or floorboards of the car. But it's my voice, and it's saying, "I'm so sorry I'm leaving you out here, Brenda."

Two weeks later, I return Brenda's lavender birthday gown, unworn (in fact, never removed from the box), to the same register at Belk where the saleswoman originally rang it up. When the new saleswoman opens the box before crediting my Visa, I'm struck again by how perfect the gown was for Brenda and how lucky I was to find it. Only one month passed between the purchase and the return.

I can see that, with time, I'll begin to free myself into my own life. The price for that freedom, though, is my sister.

Not that my old life was something to flee. There were radiant connections: A mother and father who loved me in steady ways, which is no small thing. A sister who was my portal, who showed me what was possible, ultimately showed me my own worth. Over and over, we opened ourselves wide to each other. A brother, absent early on, now a loving and loved presence. Mattie, whose tender-heartedness and care were so pure.

Maybe it's *because of* my family's closeness that we weren't able to solve the mystery of individuality and connection—how the two are in tension but also necessary to each other. How identity can be fixed, in flux, even interchangeable.

Those ties of kinship, reverberating through the generations, may have had their perils, but they also gave me something solid and lasting.

70

One Saturday, late winter, the sky was white-gold. *That bright.* Brenda and I were in our early forties. Our parents had been dead a little over a year; it would be twenty years before Brenda's diagnosis of bile duct cancer. She had called the night before, excited about a place she'd heard about: Bell's Antiques in Cleveland County, near Shelby, North Carolina, about forty-five miles from Charlotte.

"We've got to go, Judy!" she'd said. "It's supposed to be great!"

Midmorning, we headed out, each of us dreaming of bargains. I hoped to find a wicker rocker for my screened porch. Brenda still collected majolica, so she was in the market for a vase or pitcher. Also, she wouldn't mind finding an old wooden wheelbarrow decayed to grey, to plant ferns and Lenten roses in.

She was driving. I flicked on the heater, and warmth rushed to fill the car. We'd thrown our coats in the back seat. We were

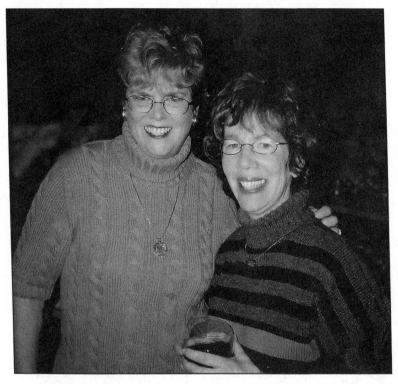

With Brenda, 2004

spinning stories about our kids, her work, my work, all the things we'd saved up to tell.

We wondered if we'd been so busy talking we missed the turnoff. Which led to kidding about how neither of us had a decent sense of direction, something we'd kidded about a million times before.

"If Chuck were with us," she said, "we'd be there."

"Oh, my gosh," I said, "Henry would know exactly how to find it. He even knows east and west."

How we loved having the exact same conversation over and over, the comforting rhythms, how it could be almost a physi-

cal expression of affection, like adjusting the other's earring and
touching her skin, too.

Down one country road, up another. We got caught behind
a slow-moving tractor because the road was hilly and we couldn't
pass. Surely, the antique store was up ahead. Finally, we spotted a
gas station still in business. A man in overalls was pumping gas.
Brenda pulled up beside him, rolled down her window, asked if
he knew where Bell's Antiques was. He did. Yes, indeed. He went
into great detail, pointing off into the distance, curving his body
to show what the road would do, counting off with his fingers
how many somethings we would pass.

Brenda thanked him, rolled her window up, pulled back onto
the road. She smiled that smile that looked so much like our father's. "I didn't understand a word he said."

"Me neither."

More laughs. All we could do was head back to the main road,
then take a side road we should've seen before but didn't.

When signs for Shelby appeared, we thought maybe we
would just follow them into town and ask there, but then we
didn't see any more signs for Shelby.

Around noon, I said, "I'm getting hungry."

"Me, too," she said. Minutes later: "There!" She pointed to
a crumbling sign on the side of the road. *B-B-Q* was all it said.
"Want to try it?"

"Sure." We both loved finding out-of-the-way places to eat.

We turned off, followed a second *B-B-Q* sign onto a dirt road,
bumped along till we came to a run-down restaurant, its wood
siding peeling, roof missing shingles, sign knocked lopsided.

In the parking lot, we reached for our coats. I was thinking,
This might be a little too out-of-the-way. I knew Brenda was thinking the same thing.

But the place was packed. A waitress, young and ponytailed,

pointed us to a table by a window that was newly washed and sparkling. She handed us paper menus and named the specials, said we'd picked a nice day to eat lunch out and were we sisters, gosh, we sounded so much alike. Yes, we answered, we are sisters, and did she know where Bell's Antiques was? She didn't. We took our time reading the menu, ordering, eating, letting ourselves fall under the spell of pork and Brunswick stew cooked just right.

Back in the car, we felt renewed and determined. We didn't even take off our coats; we were so sure we were close. We drove, talked, laughed, well into the afternoon. The light came and went. And came again.

It turned out we never did find Bell's. We'd been on the road five hours when we finally gave up and headed home. We'd been as lost as anyone could be. Yet we felt we could find our way anywhere. That's how full of love we were.